PRENATAL NUTRITION

A Self-Care Approach to Nourishing Your Body and Baby

ROSE HARPER

TABLE OF CONTENT

INTRODUCTION

In the quiet, calm spaces before the sunrise, I often found myself awake and alert, a mother on the edge of a whole new world. Back then, I was blissfully unaware that my path toward motherhood would be a journey of learning and self-discovery in more ways than one. This book, "Prenatal Nutrition: A Self-Care Approach to Nourishing Your Body and Baby," is an account of this incredibly enriching journey.

When the first signs of pregnancy set in, my life took a visible change. Morning sickness, hormonal changes, and mood swings became constant companions. As I navigated through these unfamiliar winding paths with a joyous heart, I realized that this was not just about me anymore. There was another life budding inside me, depending on me for its nutrition and survival. The onus was on me to feed two bodies mine and my baby's.

Being a first-time expectant mother, my knowledge of prenatal nutrition was limited. My journey into exploring its depths started with apprehension but soon turned into curiosity. I read research papers, reached out to professionals, and joined online forums for expectant mothers, all in an endeavor to nourish us in the best way possible. The more I learned, the more I realized how crucial proper nutrition was for my baby's development and my well-being.

Incorporating prenatal nutrition into my daily diet came with its challenges. There were foods I had to let go of and new ones I had to embrace. I swapped out caffeine for herbal teas, sugary snacks for fresh fruits, and processed foods for whole grains. Doctors' visits turned into nutrition counseling sessions, and my kitchen transformed into a sanctuary where both delicious and nutritious meals were cooked. Experimenting with new recipes and discovering nutrient-rich foods became a joyful part of my routine.

Despite the initial discomfort of change, within weeks, I observed positive outcomes. My energy levels were up, mood swings were less drastic, and even my doctor was impressed with the fetus's development. These subtle but significant improvements affirmed that I was doing something right. I felt more connected to my body and my baby, knowing that each meal was a step toward a healthier pregnancy.

Looking back at my bittersweet journey from being a clueless expectant mother to becoming a well-informed one, I cannot stress enough the importance of prenatal nutrition. It was this newfound understanding, coupled with the desire to empower other eager moms-to-be, that led me to pen down my experiences and knowledge into this book.

As you turn the pages, remember my journey is not a prescriptive diet plan but an inspiring tale. If my story nudges you toward giving the best care and nourishment to your body and baby, then I consider my purpose fulfilled. Welcome aboard on this enlightening ride toward conscious motherhood! Together, we can embrace this journey with confidence, knowing that every bite we take has the power to shape our future and the future of our little ones.

CHAPTER 1

UNDERSTANDING PRENATAL NUTRITION: THE FOUNDATIONS OF A HEALTHY PREGNANCY

As I sat in the waiting room, nervously thumbing through an old magazine, my name was finally called. Dr. Singh, with her ever-comforting smile, welcomed me into her office. "Congratulations, you're going to be a mom!" she said. And just like that, my whole world changed.

When I first discovered I was pregnant, I was overwhelmed with a mix of excitement and anxiety. There was so much to learn and so many changes to embrace. One of the first things that caught my attention was the importance of prenatal nutrition. I quickly realized that this journey wasn't just about eating more; it was about eating right.

The importance of prenatal nutrition cannot be overstated. Proper nutrition during pregnancy is crucial for the health of both the mother and the baby. For the mother, good nutrition helps maintain her energy levels, supports her body's increased demands, and prepares her for the physical challenges of childbirth. For the baby, it ensures proper growth and development, reducing the risk of congenital disabilities and promoting overall health.

The Beginning of My Nutritional Journey

My journey into understanding prenatal nutrition began with a simple visit to my obstetrician. Dr. Singh handed me a brochure and encouraged me to read it. The brochure highlighted the basics: the need for increased calories, the importance of certain vitamins and minerals, and foods to avoid. It was a lot to take in, but I was determined to give my baby the best start in life.

At first, my knowledge of prenatal nutrition was limited. I knew that folic acid was important to prevent neural tube defects, and I had heard about the importance of calcium for bone health. Beyond that, I was clueless. My curiosity led me to seek more information. I spent hours reading research papers, browsing reputable websites, and joining online forums where expectant mothers shared their experiences and advice.

The Importance of Essential Nutrients

Through my research, I learned about the essential nutrients that play critical roles during pregnancy:

Folic Acid: Vital for preventing neural tube defects, folic acid is crucial in the early weeks of pregnancy. I made sure to include foods rich in folic acid, such as leafy greens, legumes, and fortified cereals, in my diet.

Calcium: Necessary for the development of the baby's bones and teeth, calcium also helps prevent maternal bone loss. Dairy products, almonds, and leafy greens became staples in my meals.

Iron: As pregnancy increases blood volume, the need for iron rises to prevent anemia. I incorporated iron-rich foods like lean meats, beans, and spinach, and paired them with vitamin C-rich foods to enhance absorption.

Omega-3 Fatty Acids: These are crucial for the baby's brain and eye development. I added sources like salmon, flaxseeds, and walnuts to my diet.

Protein: Essential for the growth of fetal tissues, including the brain, protein also helps with the growth of the mother's uterine and breast tissue. I ensured I had enough protein from eggs, lean meats, tofu, and legumes.

Navigating Cravings and Aversions

Pregnancy brought about a rollercoaster of cravings and aversions. I remember nursing a particularly fierce craving for pickles one night and then curiously wondering how this could possibly be beneficial for my baby. I found out it is normal to have such cravings and they may not necessarily indicate nutritional deficiencies, as is commonly believed.

Food aversions were quite another thing. I made several visits to the farmers market, filling my basket with fresh fruits and veggies, only to find myself unable to stomach them later due to sudden aversions. Balancing my diet became an everyday challenge, but I learned to be flexible and adapt to my body's needs without compromising on nutrition.

Incorporating prenatal nutrition into my daily life came with its challenges. There were foods I had to let go of and new ones I had to embrace. I swapped out caffeine for herbal teas, sugary snacks for fresh fruits, and processed foods for whole grains. My kitchen transformed into a sanctuary where both delicious and nutritious meals were cooked.

A particularly enlightening conversation with a nutritionist helped me understand the crucial role of individual nutrients. For example, folic acid for neural development, calcium for bone health, and iron for increased blood volume—all played unique parts in nurturing my unborn child. This understanding empowered me to make informed decisions about my diet.

Hydration also became a priority. After a bout of dehydration landed me in the hospital, carrying a water bottle became second nature. I learned to listen to my body and respond to its needs promptly.

The journey was not always smooth sailing. Hormonal changes presented new battles every day, and I found myself daunted by the amassed myths and misconceptions surrounding prenatal nutrition. Could eating for two lead to unhealthy weight gain? Do spicy foods trigger labor? These questions were common, and I understood that taking a self-care approach required me to question, research, and make informed decisions about my diet.

One myth I encountered was the idea that pregnant women need to "eat for two." While it's true that pregnancy increases nutritional needs, it doesn't mean doubling the food intake. Instead, it's about making nutrient-dense choices. Another misconception was that cravings indicate what the body needs. While cravings are common, they don't always reflect nutritional deficiencies.

Personal Anecdotes and Experiences

My personal journey with prenatal nutrition was filled with memorable moments. I recall grocery shopping trips where I'd meticulously read labels and choose the best options for my diet. Cooking became a creative outlet, where I experimented with recipes that were both nutritious and satisfying. Meals were not just about sustenance; they were a way to connect with my growing baby and provide the best nourishment possible.

Conversations with my healthcare team were invaluable. My obstetrician and nutritionist offered practical advice and support. They emphasized the importance of balance—not just in terms of nutrients, but also in maintaining a healthy lifestyle that included physical activity and rest.

Positive Outcomes and Reflections

Despite the initial discomfort of change, within weeks, I observed positive outcomes. My energy levels were up, mood swings were less drastic, and even my doctor was impressed with the fetus's development. These subtle but significant improvements affirmed that I was doing something right. I felt more connected to my body and my baby, knowing that each meal was a step toward a healthier pregnancy.

I realized that prenatal nutrition is more than just following a dietary plan. It's about understanding your body's needs, meticulously balancing nutrient intake, navigating through cravings and aversions, and debunking myths along the way. It's a holistic approach that encompasses physical, mental, and emotional well-being.

Going into Nutrients and Their Roles

To further emphasize the importance of each nutrient, let's take a quick overview look at their specific roles and how they benefit both the mother and the baby.

Folic Acid

Folic acid, a B vitamin, is crucial during the first trimester when the neural tube is forming. The neural tube later develops into the baby's brain and spinal cord. Insufficient folic acid can lead to neural tube defects such as spina bifida. I made it a point to start my day with a breakfast rich in folic acid—fortified cereals, a glass of orange juice, and a spinach omelet.

Calcium

Calcium is not only essential for the baby's bone and teeth development but also helps in the functioning of the muscular, circulatory, and nervous systems. I ensured that my diet included a variety of calcium-rich foods like milk, yogurt, cheese, and leafy greens. I also took calcium supplements as recommended by my doctor to meet the daily requirements.

Iron

Iron is vital for making hemoglobin, the protein in red blood cells that carries oxygen to other cells. During pregnancy, the body needs more iron to supply oxygen to the baby and to make up for the increased blood volume. I included iron-rich foods like red meat, poultry, fish, and legumes in my diet. To improve absorption, I paired them with vitamin C-rich foods like citrus fruits, tomatoes, and bell peppers.

Omega-3 Fatty Acids

Omega-3 fatty acids, particularly DHA, are essential for the baby's brain and eye development. I made sure to include sources like salmon, flaxseeds, chia seeds, and walnuts in my diet. Additionally, I took a prenatal vitamin that included DHA to ensure I was getting enough of this critical nutrient.

Protein

Protein is the building block of life and is essential for the growth of fetal tissues, including the brain. It also helps with the growth of the mother's uterine and breast tissue. I aimed to include a variety of protein sources in my diet, such as eggs, lean meats, fish, tofu, beans, and nuts.

Practical Tips for a Balanced Diet

Maintaining a balanced diet during pregnancy involves more than just eating the right foods. Here are some practical tips that helped me along the way:

Meal Planning: I found it helpful to plan my meals ahead of time. This ensured that I was getting a variety of nutrients and made grocery shopping easier. I created a weekly meal plan that included a balance of fruits, vegetables, whole grains, proteins, and dairy.

Portion Control : Eating smaller, more frequent meals helped me manage my energy levels and avoid overeating. I aimed for three main meals and two to three healthy snacks throughout the day.

Hydration: Staying hydrated was crucial. I carried a water bottle everywhere and set reminders to drink water throughout the day. In addition to water, I enjoyed herbal teas and diluted fruit juices for variety.

Managing Cravings: Cravings during pregnancy are common and can vary widely. While occasional indulgences were okay, I focused on nutrient-dense options that satisfied my cravings without compromising nutrition. For example, if I craved sweets, I opted for fruits or yogurt with honey.

Dealing with Aversions: Food aversions were more challenging. I experimented with different cooking methods and flavors to make nutritious foods more palatable. Sometimes, I found that blending vegetables into soups or smoothies helped me consume essential nutrients without triggering aversions.

Including Fiber: Constipation is a common issue during pregnancy, so I made sure to include plenty of fiber-rich foods like whole grains, fruits, and vegetables in my diet. These foods not only supported digestion but also helped me feel fuller longer.

Supplementation: Despite my efforts to eat a balanced diet, prenatal vitamins were an important part of my routine. They provided additional insurance that I was meeting my nutritional needs, especially for nutrients like folic acid, iron, and calcium.

Beyond physical health, prenatal nutrition also impacted my emotional and mental well-being. Eating well gave me a sense of empowerment and reassurance that I was doing everything possible to support my baby's growth and development. It became a daily ritual of self-care and connection with my unborn child.

Conversations with Healthcare Providers

Throughout my pregnancy, I had valuable conversations with healthcare providers—obstetricians, nutritionists, and midwives—who guided and supported me on my journey. These professionals offered personalized advice, monitored my health and the baby's development, and addressed any concerns or questions I had about prenatal nutrition.

I remember one particularly enlightening conversation with a nutritionist. We discussed the importance of balancing protein, carbohydrates, and fats in each meal to ensure sustained energy levels. She emphasized the need to listen to my body and adjust my diet based on its changing needs throughout pregnancy.

Navigating Myths and Misconceptions

Prenatal nutrition is often surrounded by myths and misconceptions. During my pregnancy, I encountered many well-meaning but inaccurate pieces of advice. For instance, the notion of "eating for two" was pervasive, leading some to believe that pregnancy was a free pass to indulge in excessive eating. However, I learned that pregnancy only requires about 300 extra calories per day in the second and third trimesters, and those calories should come from nutritious sources.

Another myth was the belief that spicy foods could induce labor. While spicy foods might cause discomfort or heartburn for some pregnant women, they do not trigger labor contractions. Understanding these myths helped me make informed decisions about my diet and avoid unnecessary restrictions.

As I reflect on my journey through prenatal nutrition, I realize how much I've grown and learned along the way. What began as uncertainty and apprehension transformed into confidence and empowerment. Each day, I became more attuned to the needs of my body and my growing baby.

Prenatal nutrition became a cornerstone of my pregnancy experience—a daily commitment to nurturing and supporting new life. It taught me patience and resilience as I navigated through cravings, aversions, and hormonal changes. It showed me the profound connection between what I ate and how I felt physically, emotionally, and mentally.

Prenatal nutrition is not just about following a set of dietary guidelines; it's about embracing a holistic approach to health and well-being during pregnancy. It's about nourishing your body and your baby with intention and care, one meal at a time.

Through my journey, I've come to appreciate the importance of balance, mindfulness, and informed decision-making in prenatal nutrition. It's about listening to your body, seeking guidance from healthcare professionals, and debunking myths that may create unnecessary anxiety.

As you embark on your own journey through pregnancy, I encourage you to approach prenatal nutrition with curiosity and confidence. Educate yourself, listen to your body, and celebrate each milestone along the way. Your commitment to nurturing yourself will lay the foundation for a healthy pregnancy and a thriving baby.

Remember, you're not just eating for two; you're nourishing a beautiful journey of motherhood—one that begins with the choices you make today.

Chapter 2

*Debunking Pregnancy Diet Myths: Separating
Fact from Fiction*

Pregnancy is a unique and transformative period in a woman's life, characterized by joy, anticipation, and a myriad of changes. Alongside the physical and emotional transformations, the nutritional needs of expectant mothers become a primary focus. Unfortunately, the abundance of information available today often includes persistent myths and misconceptions about what constitutes a healthy pregnancy diet. This chapter aims to debunk these myths and replace them with evidence-based nutrition advice to ensure the well-being of both mother and baby.

When I first announced my pregnancy, I was inundated with advice from well-meaning family and friends. Suddenly, everyone had an opinion on what I should or shouldn't eat. Some of this advice was helpful, but a lot of it was conflicting and, quite frankly, overwhelming. This chapter aims to cut through the noise and debunk common pregnancy diet myths, providing evidence-based nutrition advice to help you nourish your body and your baby effectively.

The Myth of "Eating for Two"

The most enduring myths about pregnancy nutrition is the notion that pregnant women need to "eat for two." While it's true that the body requires additional nutrients to support fetal development, this does not translate to doubling caloric intake. In reality, the recommended increase is modest. During the second trimester, an additional 340 calories per day is typically sufficient, rising to about 450 calories per day in the third trimester. Overeating can lead to excessive weight gain, which is associated with gestational diabetes, hypertension, and complications during delivery.

One of the first pieces of advice I received was, "You're eating for two now!" This seemed like a dream come true, giving me the green light to indulge in all my favorite foods. However, I soon learned that this common saying is a myth.

In reality, during the first trimester, your calorie needs remain the same as they were before pregnancy. Starting in the second trimester, you only need about 350-500 extra calories per day. Overeating can lead to unnecessary weight gain, which can complicate pregnancy and delivery. Instead, focus on nutrient-dense foods that provide the vitamins and minerals both you and your baby need.

Fact: Focus on Nutrient Density

Instead of increasing portion sizes dramatically, pregnant women should prioritize nutrient-dense foods. These include lean proteins, whole grains, fruits, vegetables, and dairy products, which provide essential vitamins and minerals without excessive calories. A balanced diet supports the growing baby's needs and helps maintain the mother's health.

Seafood: Friend or Foe?

Many expectant mothers avoid all seafood fearing mercury contamination. While it is crucial to avoid high-mercury fish like king mackerel, swordfish, and tilefish, many types of seafood are safe and highly beneficial during pregnancy. Low-mercury fish such as salmon, sardines, and trout are excellent sources of omega-3 fatty acids, which are vital for fetal brain development.

"Stay away from all seafood," advised one friend, warning me about the dangers of mercury. While it's true that high levels of mercury can harm your baby's developing nervous system, not all seafood is off-limits.

Fish like salmon, sardines, and tilapia are low in mercury and high in omega-3 fatty acids, which are crucial for your baby's brain development. The key is to avoid high-mercury fish like swordfish, shark, and king mackerel. I found that incorporating safe fish into my diet not only benefited my baby but also provided a delicious and nutritious variety to my meals.

Fact: Safe Seafood Choices

The FDA and EPA recommend that pregnant women consume 8-12 ounces of low-mercury seafood per week. This intake supports cognitive and visual development in the baby. Including a variety of seafood in the diet can also provide important nutrients like vitamin D and iodine.

The Coffee Conundrum

There is a common misconception that caffeine must be entirely avoided during pregnancy. While excessive caffeine intake is linked to negative outcomes, moderate consumption is generally considered safe.

As a coffee lover, one of my biggest fears was giving up my daily cup of joe. I had heard that caffeine was a big no-no during pregnancy. However, after doing some research, I found that moderate caffeine intake is generally considered safe.

Most experts agree that up to 200 mg of caffeine per day (about one 12-ounce cup of coffee) is unlikely to harm your baby. I continued to enjoy my morning coffee, knowing that it was within safe limits and that there were many other sources of nutrients to focus on throughout the day.

Fact: Moderate Caffeine Intake is Acceptable

Research suggests that consuming up to 200 milligrams of caffeine per day (about one 12-ounce cup of coffee) is unlikely to harm the baby. It is essential to account for all sources of caffeine, including tea, chocolate, and certain medications, to stay within the safe limit. Reducing caffeine gradually can help manage withdrawal symptoms and ease the transition to lower consumption levels.

Myth: Pregnant Women Should Not Exercise

While it's true that certain high-impact or high-risk activities should be avoided during pregnancy, regular exercise is highly beneficial for most pregnant women. Exercise can help manage weight gain, reduce pregnancy-related discomfort, improve mood, and prepare the body for labor.

Activities like walking, swimming, prenatal yoga, and light strength training were a regular part of my routine. Always consult with your healthcare provider before starting any new exercise program, but know that staying active is typically a positive part of a healthy pregnancy.

Fact: Exercise is Beneficial

Regular exercise during pregnancy can improve mood, reduce discomfort, and promote overall health. Activities such as walking, swimming, and prenatal yoga are generally safe and beneficial. However, it is important to consult with a healthcare provider before starting any new exercise regimen.

The Deli Meat Debate

Another commonly heard myth is that all deli meats are off-limits due to the risk of listeria, a bacteria that can cause severe infections. While it's true that pregnant women are more susceptible to listeria, the risk can be minimized with proper handling and preparation.

Heating deli meats until steaming hot before eating can kill harmful bacteria. I found myself craving a turkey sandwich now and then, and by ensuring it was properly heated, I could satisfy my craving without worry.

Carbs: Friend or Foe?

In the age of low-carb diets, many people suggested I cut back on carbohydrates. However, during pregnancy, carbs are an essential source of energy for both you and your baby. The key is choosing the right kind of carbs.

Whole grains like brown rice, quinoa, and whole wheat bread are rich in fiber, vitamins, and minerals. These complex carbs provide sustained energy and help keep blood sugar levels stable. I focused on incorporating whole grains into my diet and found that they helped me maintain my energy levels throughout the day.

Sugar and Sweet Cravings

Pregnancy can bring about intense cravings, often for sweet treats. Some well-meaning friends suggested I indulge my cravings, while others advised against any sugar intake. The truth lies somewhere in between.

Moderation is key. Occasional treats are perfectly fine, but excessive sugar can lead to unwanted weight gain and increased risk of gestational diabetes. I allowed myself a piece of dark chocolate or a homemade cookie, balancing it with nutrient-rich meals to ensure my overall diet remained healthy.

The Organic Obsession

"Only eat organic!" a friend emphatically told me. While organic foods can reduce exposure to pesticides, they are often more expensive and not always necessary. The most important thing is to eat a variety of fruits and vegetables, whether they are organic or not.

Washing fruits and vegetables thoroughly can help remove pesticide residues. I opted for organic when it fit my budget but didn't stress if I chose conventionally grown produce. The goal was to consume a wide range of nutrients from various sources.

Dairy and Calcium

I had always enjoyed dairy products, but some friends advised against them due to concerns about hormones and antibiotics. However, dairy products are an excellent source of calcium, essential for your baby's developing bones and teeth.

Choosing organic or hormone-free dairy products can alleviate some concerns. Additionally, there are plenty of non-dairy sources of calcium, such as leafy greens, almonds, and fortified plant-based milks. I continued to enjoy dairy, supplemented by other calcium-rich foods, to ensure I was meeting my needs.

Spicy Foods and Labor

"Spicy foods can induce labor," warned a well-meaning aunt. While this myth is widespread, there's no scientific evidence to support it. Eating spicy foods can sometimes cause heartburn or indigestion, but it won't trigger labor.

I enjoyed my favorite spicy dishes in moderation, mindful of their effect on my digestion rather than any mythical labor-inducing properties.

Fact: Spicy Foods Are Generally Safe
Spicy foods do not harm the baby or cause preterm labor. However, they can cause discomfort for the mother, such as heartburn or indigestion, which are common during pregnancy. If you enjoy spicy foods and they do not cause significant discomfort, there is no need to eliminate them from your diet.

Hydration Myths

Staying hydrated is crucial during pregnancy, but the idea that you must drink a specific amount of water every day can be misleading. Individual needs vary, and factors like activity level, climate, and overall health play a role in how much water you need.

A general guideline is to drink when you're thirsty and ensure your urine is a light yellow color. I carried a water bottle with me and sipped throughout the day, focusing on staying hydrated rather than hitting an arbitrary target.

Debunking these myths helped me feel more confident in my dietary choices and less stressed about following well-intentioned but misguided advice. Here are some additional tips and insights I gathered during my pregnancy journey:

Myth: Pregnant Women Should Avoid All Herbal Teas
Herbal teas can be a comforting and healthy choice during pregnancy, but it's essential to choose wisely. Some herbs, such as raspberry leaf and peppermint, are generally

considered safe and can even help with common pregnancy symptoms like nausea and digestive issues. However, other herbs like licorice root and certain high-caffeine teas should be avoided due to potential risks.

Consulting with a healthcare provider or a knowledgeable herbalist can help you determine which teas are safe and beneficial. I found that sipping on ginger tea helped ease my morning sickness, while chamomile tea was a soothing bedtime ritual.

Myth: Cravings Indicate Nutritional Deficiencies

Many people believe that pregnancy cravings are the body's way of signaling a nutritional deficiency. While cravings can sometimes reflect a need for specific nutrients, they are more often related to hormonal changes and psychological factors.

I craved ice cream frequently, but this didn't necessarily mean I needed more calcium. Instead, I focused on maintaining a balanced diet and allowed myself to indulge cravings in moderation. Recognizing that cravings are a normal part of pregnancy helped me manage them without guilt.

Myth: All Fats Are Bad

Not all fats are created equal. Healthy fats, such as those found in avocados, nuts, seeds, and olive oil, are crucial for the development of the baby's brain and eyes. Omega-3 fatty acids, in particular, play a significant role in fetal development. Pregnant women should aim to include sources of healthy fats in their diet while limiting trans fats and saturated fats, which are found in processed and fried foods.

Fats are a vital part of a healthy diet, especially during pregnancy. Healthy fats, such as those found in avocados, nuts, seeds, and olive oil, support the development of your baby's brain and nervous system.

Trans fats and excessive saturated fats should be limited, but don't shy away from incorporating healthy fats into your meals. I found that adding avocado to my salads and snacking on nuts helped me feel satisfied and provided essential nutrients.

Pregnancy is a unique experience for every woman, and it's essential to listen to your body and consult with healthcare professionals for personalized advice. As you navigate through this special time, remember that balance, variety, and moderation are key. Trust your instincts, stay informed, and enjoy the journey of nurturing your growing baby.

Debunking these myths with evidence-based information is essential for the health and peace of mind of expecting mothers. Accurate nutritional advice ensures that both the mother and baby receive the necessary nutrients for optimal health and development. By focusing on a balanced diet rich in whole foods and essential nutrients, expectant mothers can confidently nourish their bodies and their babies.

Key Takeaways:

No need to "eat for two"; a moderate caloric increase suffices.

Certain seafood is healthy and beneficial during pregnancy, especially low-mercury options.

Cravings do not necessarily indicate nutritional needs; focus on balanced nutrition.

Healthy fats are essential for fetal development; include sources like avocados and nuts.

Moderate caffeine intake (up to 200 mg per day) is generally safe.

Many cheeses are safe if made from pasteurized milk; check labels to ensure safety.

Spicy foods are safe but may cause discomfort; eat them in moderation if they do not cause significant issues.

Calcium can be obtained from various sources, not just milk; include a variety of calcium-rich foods in your diet.

Exercise is beneficial and can improve mood, reduce discomfort, and promote overall health.

Some herbal teas are safe and can help alleviate pregnancy symptoms; consult a healthcare provider before consumption.

Practical Tips:

Meal Planning and Sample Menus: Plan meals that include a variety of nutrient-dense foods. A sample daily menu could include oatmeal with fruit for breakfast, a salad with lean protein for lunch, and grilled fish with vegetables for dinner.

Reflecting on my pregnancy journey, I realized that separating fact from fiction in prenatal nutrition is crucial for both peace of mind and health. Misinformation can lead to unnecessary stress and poor dietary choices, while evidence-based advice empowers you to nourish yourself and your baby effectively.

Chapter 3

Essential Nutrients for Pregnancy: The Role of Vitamins and Minerals

As an experienced prenatal nutritionist, I have guided many expecting mothers through their pregnancy journeys. One of the most crucial aspects of a healthy pregnancy is ensuring that both the mother and the developing baby receive adequate nutrition. This chapter of "Prenatal Nutrition: A Self-Care Approach to Nourishing Your Body and Baby" focuses on essential vitamins, minerals, and supplements necessary for a healthy pregnancy. Understanding the roles these nutrients play can help you make informed decisions about your diet and supplementation, ensuring the best possible outcomes for both you and your baby.

Vitamin D: The Sunshine Vitamin

In my years of practice as a prenatal nutritionist, I have come to appreciate the critical role of Vitamin D in pregnancy. Known as the sunshine vitamin, Vitamin D is vital for the absorption of calcium, ensuring the proper development of your baby's bones and teeth. It also plays a role in maintaining your immune system and reducing the risk of complications like preeclampsia.

I often recommend that pregnant women aim for about 600 IU of Vitamin D daily. However, depending on where you live and how much time you spend outdoors, supplementation might be necessary. Foods rich in Vitamin D include fatty fish like salmon, fortified dairy products, and egg yolks. It's always best to check with your healthcare provider to determine if you need a supplement and, if so, how much.

Iron: The Energy Enabler

Iron is another crucial nutrient during pregnancy. As your blood volume increases to support your growing baby, so does your need for iron. This mineral is essential for making hemoglobin, the protein in red blood cells that carries oxygen to your tissues and your baby. Without enough iron, you may develop anemia, which can lead to fatigue and complications such as preterm delivery.

The recommended daily intake of iron during pregnancy is about 27 mg. Iron-rich foods include lean meats, spinach, beans, and fortified cereals. In some cases, your doctor may suggest an iron supplement, especially if you're found to be anemic. Pairing iron-rich foods with vitamin C-rich foods like oranges or strawberries can enhance iron absorption.

Folate (Folic Acid): The Neural Protector

Folate, or folic acid in its synthetic form, is one of the most well-known vitamins for pregnancy. This B-vitamin is essential for the formation of the neural tube, which later develops into the baby's brain and spinal cord. Adequate folate intake can significantly reduce the risk of neural tube defects such as spina bifida.

I always advise expecting mothers to start taking 400-800 micrograms of folic acid daily, even before conception if possible, and continue throughout pregnancy. Leafy green vegetables, citrus fruits, beans, and fortified cereals are excellent sources of folate. Many prenatal vitamins also contain the necessary amount of folic acid.

Calcium: The Bone Builder

Calcium is essential for building your baby's bones and teeth, as well as ensuring your own bone health. During pregnancy, if you don't get enough calcium, your body will take it from your bones to provide for your baby, which can increase your risk of osteoporosis later in life.

Pregnant women need about 1,000 mg of calcium daily. Dairy products like milk, cheese, and yogurt are rich sources of calcium. If you're lactose intolerant or prefer non-dairy options, look for fortified plant-based milks and juices, as well as calcium-rich foods like tofu, almonds, and leafy green vegetables.

Omega-3 Fatty Acids: The Brain Boosters

Omega-3 fatty acids, particularly DHA (docosahexaenoic acid), play a crucial role in the development of your baby's brain and eyes. They are also beneficial for reducing the risk of preterm birth and promoting a healthy birth weight.

Aim for at least 200-300 mg of DHA daily. Fatty fish like salmon, mackerel, and sardines are excellent sources of omega-3s. If you're not a fan of fish or if you're vegetarian or vegan, you can find DHA supplements derived from algae. Many prenatal vitamins now include DHA to help you meet your needs.

Vitamin C: The Immune Supporter

Vitamin C is essential for the growth and repair of tissues in both you and your baby. It also helps your body absorb iron more efficiently, which is particularly important during pregnancy. Additionally, Vitamin C supports your immune system and may help reduce the risk of developing complications such as preeclampsia.

The recommended daily intake of Vitamin C during pregnancy is about 85 mg. Citrus fruits like oranges, grapefruits, and lemons are well-known sources, but you can also find Vitamin C in strawberries, bell peppers, broccoli, and tomatoes. Most prenatal vitamins contain adequate amounts of Vitamin C, ensuring you get enough of this crucial nutrient.

Vitamin A: The Vision and Immunity Booster

Vitamin A is essential for your baby's vision, immune function, and cell growth. However, it's important to get the right balance, as too much preformed Vitamin A (found in animal products and some supplements) can be harmful.

During pregnancy, you need about 770 micrograms of Vitamin A daily. It's best to get this from a combination of sources, including beta-carotene (found in colorful fruits and vegetables like carrots, sweet potatoes, and spinach) and preformed Vitamin A (found in animal products like liver and dairy). Always consult your healthcare provider before taking Vitamin A supplements to ensure you're within the safe range.

Vitamin B6: The Nausea Reliever

Vitamin B6, or pyridoxine, is essential for your baby's brain and nervous system development. It also helps alleviate nausea and morning sickness, which is a common complaint during the first trimester.

Pregnant women need about 1.9 mg of Vitamin B6 daily. You can find this vitamin in foods like poultry, fish, potatoes, bananas, and fortified cereals. If you're experiencing severe morning sickness, your healthcare provider might recommend a Vitamin B6 supplement to help manage your symptoms.

Vitamin B12: The Red Blood Cell Producer

Vitamin B12 is crucial for the production of red blood cells and the development of your baby's nervous system. It's particularly important for pregnant women who follow vegetarian or vegan diets, as B12 is primarily found in animal products.

The recommended daily intake of Vitamin B12 during pregnancy is 2.6 micrograms. Sources include meat, fish, dairy products, and fortified cereals. If you're not getting enough from your diet, your healthcare provider may suggest a B12 supplement to ensure you and your baby are adequately nourished.

Iodine: The Thyroid Regulator

Iodine is essential for the production of thyroid hormones, which regulate your baby's growth and brain development. During pregnancy, your need for iodine increases, and inadequate intake can lead to developmental delays and other complications.

Pregnant women need about 220 micrograms of iodine daily. Good dietary sources include iodized salt, dairy products, seafood, and eggs. If you're not consuming enough iodine-rich foods, a supplement may be necessary. Always consult your healthcare provider to determine if supplementation is right for you.

Magnesium: The Muscle and Nerve Supporter

Magnesium is important for numerous bodily functions, including muscle and nerve function, blood sugar regulation, and bone development. During pregnancy, adequate magnesium intake can help prevent complications such as preterm labor and preeclampsia. The recommended daily intake of magnesium during pregnancy is about 350-360 mg. You can find magnesium in foods like nuts, seeds, whole grains, and leafy green vegetables. If your diet doesn't provide enough magnesium, your healthcare provider may suggest a supplement to ensure you meet your needs.

Zinc: The Cell Growth Facilitator

Zinc is crucial for cell growth, immune function, and DNA synthesis. During pregnancy, it supports the rapid cell growth that occurs in your developing baby and helps maintain your immune system.

Pregnant women need about 11 mg of zinc daily. Good dietary sources include meat, shellfish, legumes, seeds, and nuts. If you're not getting enough zinc from your diet, your healthcare provider may recommend a supplement to ensure you and your baby are adequately supported.

Choline: The Brain and Spinal Cord Developer

Choline is essential for the development of your baby's brain and spinal cord. It also helps prevent neural tube defects and supports your body's metabolism.

Pregnant women need about 450 mg of choline daily. You can find choline in foods like eggs, meat, fish, dairy products, and some nuts and beans. If your diet doesn't provide enough choline, your healthcare provider may suggest a supplement to ensure you meet your needs.

Each vitamin and mineral plays a unique role in supporting your health and your baby's development. Remember, it's always best to consult with your healthcare provider or a dietitian before making any changes to your diet or supplement regimen. Every pregnancy is unique, and your healthcare team can provide personalized advice to ensure you and your baby are getting the nutrients you need.

In my experience, focusing on a varied diet rich in fruits, vegetables, lean proteins, and whole grains can help you meet most of your nutritional needs. However, prenatal vitamins and supplements can be valuable tools to fill any gaps and support a healthy pregnancy. Your journey to nourish your body and baby is a vital one, and understanding the role of these essential nutrients is a key step in that journey.

The Role of Macronutrients in Pregnancy

In addition to vitamins and minerals, macronutrients play a crucial role in supporting a healthy pregnancy. Proteins, carbohydrates, and fats provide the energy and building blocks needed for the growth and development of your baby.

Proteins are essential for the growth of fetal tissue, including the brain. They also help increase your blood supply, allowing more blood to be sent to your baby. Aim for about 75-100 grams of protein per day from sources like lean meats, eggs, dairy products, beans, and nuts.

Carbohydrates are your body's primary energy source. They provide the energy needed to support the increased metabolic demands of pregnancy. Focus on complex carbohydrates like whole grains, fruits, and vegetables to maintain steady energy levels and support digestive health.

Fats, particularly omega-3 fatty acids, are vital for brain development and the formation of cell membranes. Include healthy fats from sources like avocados, nuts, seeds, and fatty fish in your diet.

Hydration and Pregnancy

Staying hydrated is essential for maintaining your health and supporting your baby's development. During pregnancy, your body needs more fluids to form amniotic fluid, produce extra blood, build new tissue, carry nutrients, and help in digestion.

Aim to drink at least 8-10 glasses of water daily. Remember that other fluids like herbal teas, milk, and fruit juices also contribute to your hydration needs. Proper hydration helps prevent common pregnancy issues like constipation, urinary tract infections, and swelling.

Common Nutritional Deficiencies and How to Address Them

During pregnancy, certain nutritional deficiencies are more common and can have serious consequences if not addressed.

Iron deficiency can lead to anemia, causing fatigue and increasing the risk of preterm birth. Ensure you consume iron-rich foods and consider supplementation if necessary.

Calcium deficiency can affect your baby's bone development and increase the risk of osteoporosis in mothers. Include dairy products or fortified plant-based alternatives in your diet.

Vitamin D deficiency is linked to complications like preeclampsia and gestational diabetes. Ensure adequate sun exposure and include vitamin D-rich foods or supplements in your routine.

Regular prenatal check-ups can help monitor your nutritional status and prevent deficiencies. Your healthcare provider may recommend specific supplements or dietary adjustments based on your individual needs.

The Impact of Nutrition on Pregnancy Complications

Proper nutrition can play a significant role in preventing or managing pregnancy complications. For instance, a balanced diet rich in fiber can help prevent gestational diabetes by regulating blood sugar levels. Similarly, adequate calcium and vitamin D intake can reduce the risk of preeclampsia, a condition characterized by high blood pressure and organ damage.

Maintaining a healthy weight through proper nutrition and regular exercise can also lower the risk of complications. Consult with your healthcare provider to develop a nutrition plan tailored to your needs and monitor your progress throughout your pregnancy.

Dietary Supplements and Their Safety

While a balanced diet is the best way to obtain essential nutrients, dietary supplements can help fill any gaps. Prenatal vitamins typically contain a mix of essential vitamins and minerals, including folic acid, iron, calcium, and DHA.

It's important to choose supplements that are specifically designed for pregnancy and to follow your healthcare provider's recommendations regarding dosage. Avoid taking additional supplements without professional guidance, as excessive intake of certain nutrients can be harmful.

Meal Planning and Nutritional Tips for Pregnant Women
Planning nutritious meals can help ensure you and your baby receive the necessary nutrients. Aim for a variety of foods from all food groups to create a balanced diet.

Breakfast: Start your day with a meal rich in protein and fiber, such as a smoothie with Greek yogurt, spinach, and berries, or whole-grain toast with avocado and a boiled egg.

Lunch: Include a variety of vegetables, lean protein, and whole grains. A quinoa salad with grilled chicken, mixed greens, and a vinaigrette dressing is a great option.

Dinner: Focus on lean proteins, vegetables, and healthy fats. Consider baked salmon with sweet potatoes and steamed broccoli.

Snacks: Keep healthy snacks on hand, such as nuts, fruits, and yogurt, to maintain energy levels throughout the day.

Nutritional Considerations for Special Diets
If you follow a special diet, such as vegetarian, vegan, or gluten-free, it's important to ensure you still get all the essential nutrients.

For vegetarians and vegans, focus on plant-based sources of protein, iron, calcium, and vitamin B12. Consider fortified foods and supplements to meet your needs.

For those on a gluten-free diet, choose whole grains like quinoa, rice, and gluten-free oats to ensure adequate fiber and nutrient intake. Pay attention to fortified gluten-free products to avoid deficiencies.

The Importance of Regular Prenatal Check-ups

Regular prenatal check-ups are vital for monitoring your health and your baby's development. Your healthcare provider can help track your nutritional status, recommend appropriate supplements, and adjust your diet as needed.

These check-ups also provide an opportunity to discuss any concerns you may have about your diet or any symptoms you're experiencing. By staying proactive about your nutrition, you can help ensure a healthy pregnancy for you and your baby.

The Influence of Lifestyle Factors on Prenatal Nutrition

Lifestyle factors such as stress, physical activity, and sleep can significantly impact your nutritional needs during pregnancy. Managing stress through relaxation techniques, maintaining a moderate exercise routine, and ensuring adequate sleep can all contribute to better nutritional status and overall health.

Engage in activities like prenatal yoga, meditation, and gentle walking to support your physical and mental well-being. Aim for 7-9 hours of sleep each night and create a relaxing bedtime routine to improve sleep quality.

Cultural Perspectives on Prenatal Nutrition

Different cultures have unique approaches to prenatal nutrition, often incorporating traditional foods and practices that support a healthy pregnancy. Exploring these perspectives can provide valuable insights and diversify your dietary options.

For example, traditional Japanese diets include nutrient-rich foods like fish, seaweed, and fermented products, which offer essential omega-3 fatty acids and probiotics. Indian cuisine often features lentils, vegetables, and spices like turmeric, which provide a wealth of vitamins, minerals, and anti-inflammatory properties.

Incorporating a variety of cultural foods into your diet can enhance your nutrient intake and add variety to your meals. Always consider your dietary preferences and consult with your healthcare provider before making significant changes.

Pregnancy is a time of increased nutritional demands, and ensuring you receive adequate vitamins, minerals, and supplements is crucial for both your health and your baby's development. From the essential roles of vitamins and minerals to the importance of macronutrients and hydration, each aspect of prenatal nutrition plays a vital role in supporting a healthy pregnancy.

By focusing on a balanced diet rich in essential nutrients, staying hydrated, and consulting with your healthcare provider for personalized guidance, you can help ensure the best possible outcomes for you and your baby. Remember, every pregnancy is unique, and your nutritional needs may vary. Always seek professional advice before making significant dietary changes or starting new supplements.

With the right knowledge and support, you can nourish your body and your baby for a healthy, happy pregnancy journey.

Chapter 4

*First Trimester Nutrition: Laying the Groundwork
for a Healthy Start*

In this beautiful path of motherhood, I realized that the first trimester is not just about dealing with morning sickness. It's about laying the groundwork for our baby's health and development. During these initial weeks, the foundations for vital organs, the nervous system, and the brain are being formed. Proper nutrition is essential for supporting these rapid developments and ensuring that both mother and baby are healthy.

During my first trimester, I discovered that focusing on nutrient-dense foods was critical. Eating a variety of fruits, vegetables, whole grains, lean proteins, and healthy fats provided the essential nutrients needed for this crucial stage. These foods are packed with vitamins, minerals, and antioxidants that support both the baby's growth and my well-being.

Frequently Asked Questions (FAQ)

When I first found out I was pregnant, I was flooded with excitement and a million questions, especially about what I should and shouldn't be eating. The first trimester can be particularly overwhelming with all the changes happening in your body and the wealth of information out there. I spent countless hours researching and asking my doctor questions to make sure I was doing everything right for my baby and myself. To help other moms-to-be navigate this crucial period, I've compiled some of the most frequently asked questions about first trimester nutrition that I encountered along the way. These answers are based on what I learned and my own experiences. I hope they provide the reassurance and clarity you're looking for.

Can I drink coffee during my first trimester?

One of the first things I worried about was my morning coffee. I learned that you can still enjoy coffee, but moderation is key. Experts recommend limiting caffeine intake to about 200 milligrams per day, which is roughly one 12-ounce cup. Too much caffeine can increase the risk of miscarriage and low birth weight, so I made sure to stick to one cup and enjoyed it even more knowing it was safe.

What are the best foods to eat if I'm experiencing morning sickness?

Morning sickness hit me hard, and finding foods that didn't make me feel worse was a challenge. I discovered that eating small, frequent meals helped manage the nausea. Bland, easy-to-digest foods like crackers, toast, bananas, and applesauce were lifesavers. Ginger and peppermint also worked wonders in soothing my stomach.

Do I need to take prenatal vitamins?

Yes, prenatal vitamins are essential. I started taking them as soon as I found out I was pregnant. They fill in the nutritional gaps and ensure you and your baby get vital nutrients like folic acid, iron, and calcium. Your healthcare provider can help you choose the right prenatal vitamin for you.

Are there any foods I should avoid during the first trimester?

I was surprised by some of the foods I had to steer clear of. High-mercury fish like shark and swordfish were off the menu, as well as raw or undercooked seafood and meat, unpasteurized dairy products, and certain deli meats and soft cheeses. These foods can pose risks to your developing baby, so I made sure to avoid them.

How much weight should I gain during the first trimester?

I was concerned about weight gain, but my doctor reassured me that it varies from woman to woman. Typically, a gain of 1-4 pounds during the first trimester is normal. Rather than focusing on the scale, I concentrated on eating a balanced diet to nourish my baby and myself.

How can I ensure I'm getting enough nutrients if I have food aversions?

Food aversions were another hurdle. When certain foods were unappealing, I found alternatives to ensure I was still getting the necessary nutrients. For example, if meat was a no-go, I opted for plant-based proteins like beans, lentils, and tofu. Smoothies became a great way to sneak in fruits and vegetables.

I hope these answers help you feel more confident and informed about your first trimester nutrition. Remember, every pregnancy is unique, so always consult with your healthcare provider for personalized advice.

Balancing Macronutrients: Proteins, Fats, and Carbs

Every bite matters now! In my experience, focusing on proteins, carbs, and healthy fats helped me nurture my growing baby.

Proteins:

Protein is vital for the growth and repair of tissues, making it crucial for both the mother and the developing baby. Good sources of protein include lean meats, poultry, fish, eggs, dairy products, beans, and legumes. I found that incorporating a variety of these foods into my meals helped me meet the recommended daily intake of 70-100 grams of protein.

Carbohydrates:

Carbohydrates provide the energy needed to support pregnancy. However, not all carbs are created equal. Complex carbohydrates, such as whole grains, fruits, and vegetables, are preferable because they release energy slowly and are packed with fiber, which aids digestion and prevents constipation – a common issue during pregnancy. I made sure to include oatmeal, brown rice, quinoa, and plenty of fresh produce in my diet.

Fats:

Healthy fats are essential for fetal brain development. Omega-3 fatty acids, found in fish like salmon, flaxseeds, chia seeds, and walnuts, are particularly important. Including these in my diet ensured that I was getting the necessary fats without overindulging in unhealthy options like Trans fats and excessive saturated fats.

Essential Micronutrients: Iron, Calcium, Folate, and More

Trust me when I say - these tiny nutrients have a giant role! When I started focusing on iron-rich foods, leafy greens, and fortified cereals, I noticed a significant improvement in my energy levels.

Folate (Folic Acid):

Folate is perhaps the most critical nutrient during the first trimester. It helps prevent neural tube defects, which can affect the brain and spine of the developing baby. I took a prenatal vitamin that included 400-600 micrograms of folic acid and ate foods rich in folate, such as leafy greens, citrus fruits, beans, and fortified cereals.

Iron:

Iron supports the increased blood volume during pregnancy and prevents anemia. I incorporated iron-rich foods like red meat, poultry, fish, lentils, and spinach. Pairing these with vitamin C-rich foods, like oranges or bell peppers, enhanced iron absorption.

Calcium:

Calcium is crucial for the development of the baby's bones and teeth. To meet the daily requirement of 1,000 milligrams, I included dairy products like milk, yogurt, and cheese, as well as non-dairy sources like fortified plant-based milks, broccoli, and almonds.

Vitamin D:

Vitamin D works hand-in-hand with calcium to support bone health. I made sure to get some sunlight exposure and included vitamin D-rich foods like fatty fish, fortified dairy, and eggs in my diet.

The Role of Hydration

Hydration plays a crucial role during the first trimester of pregnancy, supporting both maternal and fetal health. Increased blood volume, amniotic fluid production, and overall cellular functions rely heavily on adequate fluid intake. Staying well-hydrated helps to ensure that nutrients are efficiently transported to the developing baby and assists in the elimination of waste products from the mother's body.

Proper hydration can also alleviate common pregnancy-related issues such as constipation, headaches, and fatigue. During my first trimester, I made it a habit to carry a water bottle wherever I went, ensuring I sipped water throughout the day. The general recommendation is to drink at least eight to ten 8-ounce glasses of water daily, though individual needs may vary.

To maintain adequate hydration, I incorporated hydrating foods like cucumbers, watermelon, oranges, and strawberries into my diet. These fruits and vegetables not only provided additional fluids but also essential vitamins and minerals. Herbal teas and clear broths were also great additions to my hydration routine.

Recognizing signs of dehydration is crucial. Symptoms such as dark yellow urine, dry mouth, dizziness, and infrequent urination can indicate insufficient fluid intake. If you notice these signs, it's important to increase your water consumption immediately.

A practical tip I found helpful was setting reminders on my phone to drink water at regular intervals. Investing in a water bottle with marked time goals can also serve as a visual cue to keep drinking throughout the day. By prioritizing hydration, you support your body's increased demands during pregnancy and promote a healthy environment for your baby's growth and development.

Foods to Avoid During Early Pregnancy

Turning into a human shield for my little one also meant steering clear of certain foods during the first trimester. Avoiding potentially harmful foods can protect both the mother and the developing baby from risks like foodborne illnesses and exposure to harmful substances.

Raw or Undercooked Foods:I avoided raw fish (like sushi), undercooked meat, and eggs to reduce the risk of infections such as listeria, salmonella, and toxoplasmosis. Ensuring that all meats were cooked to a safe internal temperature was a must.

Unpasteurized Dairy Products:

Unpasteurized milk and cheeses can contain harmful bacteria. I checked labels to ensure that any dairy products I consumed were pasteurized.

High-Mercury Fish:

Some fish contain high levels of mercury, which can affect the baby's developing nervous system. I avoided fish like shark, swordfish, king mackerel, and tilefish, opting instead for low-mercury options like salmon, sardines, and trout.

Caffeine:

Moderating caffeine intake is important during pregnancy. I limited my caffeine consumption to 200 milligrams per day, which is about one 12-ounce cup of coffee. This helped reduce the risk of miscarriage and low birth weight.

Tips for Dealing with Morning Sickness and Food Aversions
Oh, the infamous morning sickness! Here are some tricks that helped me keep meals down and manage food aversions.

Eating Small, Frequent Meals:
Eating smaller, more frequent meals helped keep nausea at bay and maintained steady blood sugar levels. I found that having a few crackers or a piece of toast before getting out of bed in the morning helped ease the nausea.

Avoiding Strong Odors:

Certain smells triggered my nausea, so I tried to avoid cooking strong-smelling foods. Instead, I opted for bland, easy-to-digest meals like plain rice, applesauce, and toast.

Ginger and Peppermint:

Ginger and peppermint are known for their anti-nausea properties. Ginger tea, ginger candies, or peppermint tea were lifesavers during those queasy moments.

Meal Plans for Optimal Nutrient Intake

I'm excited to share some meal plans that helped me meet nutritional goals while satisfying those crazy cravings. Here are a few examples of nutrient-dense meals that are easy to prepare and enjoy during the first trimester.

Breakfast:

Option 1: Greek yogurt with fresh berries, a sprinkle of granola, and a drizzle of honey.

Option 2: Whole-grain toast with avocado and a poached egg, served with a side of sliced tomatoes.

Option 3: Smoothie made with spinach, banana, almond milk, chia seeds, and a scoop of protein powder.

Lunch:

Option 1: Quinoa salad with mixed greens, chickpeas, cherry tomatoes, cucumber, and a lemon-tahini dressing.

Option 2: Grilled chicken wrap with whole-wheat tortilla, hummus, shredded carrots, and spinach.

Option 3: Lentil soup with a side of whole-grain bread and a mixed green salad.

Dinner:

Option 1: Baked salmon with a side of roasted sweet potatoes and steamed broccoli.

Option 2: Stir-fried tofu with mixed vegetables and brown rice.

Option 3: Turkey meatballs with whole-grain pasta and a marinara sauce, served with a side of sautéed spinach.

Snacks:

Option 1: Apple slices with almond butter.

Option 2: Carrot sticks with hummus.

Option 3: Cottage cheese with pineapple chunks.

Key Points to note:

- Focus on nutrient-dense foods to support early development.
- Balance macronutrients: proteins, healthy fats, and complex carbohydrates.
- Ensure adequate intake of essential micronutrients like folate, iron, calcium, and vitamin D.
- Avoid potentially harmful foods like raw or undercooked foods, unpasteurized dairy products, and high-mercury fish.
- Manage morning sickness and food aversions with small, frequent meals, staying hydrated, and using ginger or peppermint.
- Incorporate balanced meal plans to meet nutritional needs while satisfying cravings.

Embracing this journey with a focus on self-care and nutrition will set the stage for a healthy pregnancy and a healthy baby. Don't forget to consult with your healthcare provider for personalized advice and guidance.

Chapter 5

Nourishing Growth and Preparation:

Second and Third Trimester Nutrition

Understanding pregnancy nutrition is integral to healthier birth outcomes, and the second and third trimesters are critical periods for ensuring proper nourishment for both mother and child. This chapter, "Nourishing Growth and Preparation: Second and Third Trimester Nutrition," delves into the specific dietary demands of these stages, enlightening readers on essential nutrients, meal planning, and mitigating potential health conditions through optimal prenatal nutrition.

The second trimester, spanning from weeks 13 to 26, marks a period of rapid fetal growth and significant maternal physiological changes. It is essential to focus on adequate intake of calories, protein, vitamins, and minerals to support this growth. This section will explore the specific nutrients required for sustained fetal development and maternal health, and offer practical advice on optimizing nutrition to manage conditions like gestational diabetes and anemia.

The third trimester, from weeks 27 to 40, is a time of final fetal maturation and preparation for labor and delivery. Nutritional needs peak during this period, demanding heightened attention to diet to ensure the baby receives crucial nutrients for brain development and immune function. This part of the chapter will provide detailed dietary guidelines to prepare for childbirth and postpartum recovery, emphasizing foods rich in vital nutrients.

By understanding the pivotal nutrition roles in the second and third trimesters, mothers-to-be can equip themselves with the knowledge necessary to make informed dietary decisions, fostering healthier outcomes for themselves and their babies. This comprehensive guide offers evidence-based recommendations, practical meal plans, and snack ideas to support a healthy pregnancy journey.

Second Trimester Nutrition (Week 13-26)

Nutritional Requirements for Sustained Fetal Growth and Development

During the second trimester, the fetus undergoes rapid growth and development, making proper nutrition essential for this critical phase. Key nutrients are necessary to support this growth, including an increased intake of calories, protein, vitamins, and minerals. An additional 340 calories per day are recommended to support the growing fetus, ensuring the energy demands are met without compromising maternal health.

Protein intake should be around 71 grams per day, as it is vital for tissue growth and development. Lean meats, dairy products, beans, and nuts are excellent sources of high-quality protein that can help meet these needs. Iron is another crucial nutrient during the second trimester, with a recommended intake of 27 mg per day. This increase supports the expanding blood volume and helps prevent maternal anemia. Iron-rich foods include lean red meat, poultry, fish, lentils, spinach, and fortified cereals.

Calcium intake should be 1,000 mg per day to support the development of the fetal skeleton. Dairy products, fortified plant-based milks, leafy greens, and tofu are excellent sources of calcium. Folate is another vital nutrient, with a daily recommendation of 600 mcg to help prevent neural tube defects. Leafy greens, citrus fruits, beans, and fortified cereals are good sources of folate.

Omega-3 fatty acids, particularly DHA and EPA, are important for fetal brain development. Fatty fish such as salmon and sardines, as well as flaxseeds, chia seeds, and walnuts, are rich in these fatty acids. Ensuring an adequate intake of these key nutrients can significantly contribute to the sustained growth and development of the fetus during the second trimester, laying a solid foundation for the baby's health.

Maternal Health and Energy Needs

The second trimester sees significant changes in the mother's body, requiring adjustments in dietary intake to support both maternal health and fetal growth. One of the primary changes is an increase in the mother's overall metabolism, which necessitates a higher caloric intake. An additional 340 calories per day helps sustain both maternal energy levels and fetal development, ensuring that the mother has enough energy to cope with the physical demands of pregnancy.

A balanced diet rich in whole grains, lean proteins, fruits, vegetables, and healthy fats is crucial during this period. Whole grains provide essential carbohydrates that are a primary energy source, while lean proteins support tissue growth and repair. Fruits and vegetables are rich in vitamins, minerals, and antioxidants that protect against oxidative stress and support overall health. Healthy fats, such as those found in avocados, nuts, and olive oil, are important for brain development and maintaining cellular integrity.

Hydration is another critical aspect of maternal health during the second trimester. Adequate water intake is vital for maintaining amniotic fluid levels and supporting the increased blood volume. It is recommended that pregnant women aim for at least 8-10 cups of water per day, more if they are physically active or live in hot climates.

Additionally, the second trimester is a time when many women experience relief from early pregnancy symptoms such as nausea and fatigue, making it easier to maintain a nutritious diet. However, it is also a period when some women may experience heartburn or indigestion. Eating smaller, more frequent meals and avoiding spicy or fatty foods can help manage these symptoms.

By focusing on these dietary adjustments and maintaining a balanced intake of essential nutrients, mothers can support their own health and energy needs, ensuring they have the strength and vitality to nurture their growing babies.

Optimizing Prenatal Nutrition for Specific Health Conditions
Pregnancy can present unique health challenges, such as gestational diabetes, preeclampsia, and anemia. Proper nutrition plays a crucial role in managing these conditions and ensuring both maternal and fetal health.

For mothers diagnosed with gestational diabetes, controlling carbohydrate intake and maintaining balanced blood sugar levels is essential. A diet focused on complex carbohydrates, such as whole grains, vegetables, and legumes, can help regulate blood glucose levels. It's important to avoid high-sugar foods and beverages, opting instead for nutrient-dense options that provide sustained energy without causing spikes in blood sugar. Regular monitoring of blood glucose levels and working with a healthcare provider to adjust the diet as needed is also crucial.

Preeclampsia, characterized by high blood pressure and protein in the urine, can be managed in part through dietary choices. Increasing the intake of calcium and magnesium has been shown to help reduce the risk of preeclampsia. Foods rich in these minerals include dairy products, leafy greens, nuts, seeds, and whole grains. Additionally, maintaining a balanced diet low in processed foods and high in fruits and vegetables can support overall cardiovascular health and help manage blood pressure.

Anemia, commonly caused by iron deficiency, requires an increased intake of iron to support the growing blood volume and prevent maternal and fetal complications. Incorporating iron-rich foods such as lean red meat, poultry, fish, lentils, spinach, and fortified cereals into the diet is essential. Vitamin C enhances iron absorption, so pairing iron-rich foods with vitamin C sources like citrus fruits, bell peppers, and strawberries can improve iron levels. In some cases, iron supplements may be necessary, and should be taken under the guidance of a healthcare provider.

By optimizing prenatal nutrition to address these specific health conditions, expectant mothers can manage their symptoms and support their health and the health of their babies. Tailoring dietary choices to individual health needs ensures that both mother and child receive the necessary nutrients for a healthy pregnancy.

Practical Meal Planning and Snack Ideas
Balancing nutritional needs during the second trimester can be achieved with thoughtful meal planning that incorporates essential nutrients. Practical meal and snack ideas can help ensure that both mother and baby receive the necessary nourishment without feeling overwhelmed.

For breakfast, consider starting the day with Greek yogurt topped with fresh berries and a sprinkle of flaxseeds. This combination provides a good mix of protein, calcium, antioxidants, and omega-3 fatty acids. Another option could be a smoothie made with spinach, banana, almond milk, and a scoop of protein powder, offering a nutrient-packed start to the day.

Lunch should focus on a balance of lean protein, whole grains, and vegetables. A quinoa salad with grilled chicken, mixed greens, avocado, and a lemon vinaigrette is both nutritious and satisfying. Alternatively, a lentil soup paired with whole-grain bread and a side salad can provide a hearty and nutrient-dense meal.

Dinner can be a time to include a variety of food groups. Baked salmon with roasted sweet potatoes and steamed broccoli offers a balanced meal rich in omega-3 fatty acids, vitamins, and minerals. Another option could be a stir-fry with tofu, colorful bell peppers, snap peas, and brown rice, providing a plant-based source of protein and a variety of vitamins and antioxidants.

Snacks are an important part of maintaining energy levels and preventing overeating at main meals. Healthy snack ideas include apple slices with almond butter, which offer fiber, healthy fats, and protein. Carrot sticks with hummus provide a crunchy and satisfying snack rich in vitamins and protein. A handful of mixed nuts can also be a convenient and nutrient-dense option.

Incorporating a variety of foods and maintaining a balanced diet through practical meal planning can help meet the nutritional needs of the second trimester. By focusing on whole foods and nutrient-dense options, expectant mothers can ensure they are providing the best possible nutrition for themselves and their growing babies.

Dietary Considerations for Preparation for Labor and Delivery

As the third trimester progresses, preparing for labor and delivery becomes increasingly important. Proper nutrition during this period can support maternal strength, stamina, and overall health, ensuring a smoother labor and recovery process. Key dietary considerations include maintaining hydration, balancing macronutrient intake, and focusing on specific nutrients that can aid in labor preparation.

Hydration is vital during the third trimester to support the increased blood volume and amniotic fluid levels. Adequate water intake can also help prevent common issues such as constipation and urinary tract infections. Pregnant women should aim to drink at least 8-10 cups of water daily, and more if they are physically active or live in hot climates. Including hydrating foods such as cucumbers, watermelon, and oranges in the diet can also contribute to overall hydration.

A balanced intake of carbohydrates, proteins, and fats is crucial during the third trimester. Carbohydrates provide the necessary energy for the physically demanding labor process, while proteins support tissue repair and growth. Healthy fats are important for maintaining cellular health and supporting hormone production. Whole grains, lean meats, dairy products, nuts, seeds, and avocados are excellent sources of these macronutrients.

Certain nutrients play a specific role in labor preparation. Iron continues to be essential to prevent anemia and ensure adequate oxygen supply to both mother and baby. Foods rich in iron, such as lean red meat, poultry, beans, and fortified cereals, should be included in the diet. Additionally, vitamin C can enhance iron absorption, so pairing iron-rich foods with vitamin C sources like citrus fruits and bell peppers is beneficial.

Calcium and magnesium are important for muscle function and can help prevent muscle cramps during pregnancy. Dairy products, leafy greens, nuts, and seeds are good sources of these minerals. B vitamins, particularly B6 and B12, support energy metabolism and red blood cell production, and can be found in whole grains, eggs, and dairy products.

By focusing on these dietary considerations, expectant mothers can better prepare their bodies for the demands of labor and delivery, supporting a smoother and healthier birth experience.

Nutrients and Foods Supporting Fetal Brain Development and Immune System

The third trimester is a critical period for fetal brain development and the maturation of the immune system. Proper nutrition during this stage is essential to support these processes and ensure optimal outcomes for the baby's health. Key nutrients and foods play a significant role in promoting brain development and strengthening the immune system.

Omega-3 fatty acids, particularly DHA (docosahexaenoic acid), are crucial for fetal brain development. DHA is a major structural component of the brain and retina, and adequate intake is associated with better cognitive and visual outcomes for the baby. Fatty fish such as salmon, sardines, and mackerel are rich sources of DHA. For those who do not consume fish, DHA supplements derived from algae can be an alternative.

Choline is another important nutrient for brain development. It supports the formation of the brain's structural components and the development of memory functions. Eggs are an excellent source of choline, with one egg providing about 147 mg. Pregnant women should aim for at least 450 mg of choline per day, which can be achieved through eggs, lean meats, fish, and beans.

Iron is essential for brain development and the formation of healthy neural pathways. Iron deficiency during pregnancy can lead to impaired cognitive development in the baby. Foods rich in iron, such as lean red meat, poultry, fish, lentils, and fortified cereals, should be included in the diet. Pairing iron-rich foods with vitamin C sources can enhance iron absorption.

For immune system support, vitamins A, C, and E, along with zinc, play vital roles. Vitamin A supports the development of the baby's organs and immune system. Carrots, sweet potatoes, and dark leafy greens are good sources of vitamin A. Vitamin C helps protect against infections and supports the production of collagen, which is important for the skin, blood vessels, and connective tissues. Citrus fruits, strawberries, bell peppers, and broccoli are rich in vitamin C.

Vitamin E acts as an antioxidant, protecting cells from damage. Nuts, seeds, and vegetable oils are excellent sources of vitamin E. Zinc is crucial for immune function and cellular growth, and can be found in meat, shellfish, legumes, and seeds.

By focusing on these key nutrients and incorporating a variety of nutrient-dense foods, expectant mothers can support their baby's brain development and immune system, laying a strong foundation for their child's future health.

Maternal Nutrition for Energy, Strength, and Postpartum Recovery

The third trimester is not only about preparing for the birth of the baby but also for the mother's postpartum recovery. Proper nutrition during this period can significantly impact maternal energy levels, strength, and the body's ability to recover after delivery. Key nutrients and dietary strategies can support these needs, ensuring the mother is well-prepared for the demands of childbirth and the postpartum period.

Iron remains a critical nutrient in the third trimester. The increased blood volume and the demands of childbirth can deplete iron stores, leading to anemia if not properly managed. Consuming iron-rich foods such as lean red meat, poultry, fish, lentils, spinach, and fortified cereals is essential. Pairing these foods with vitamin C sources like citrus fruits and bell peppers can enhance iron absorption and help maintain adequate iron levels.

Protein is another vital nutrient for maternal strength and recovery. Protein supports tissue repair, muscle strength, and overall energy levels. Pregnant women should aim for about 71 grams of protein per day. Good sources of protein include lean meats, fish, eggs, dairy products, beans, nuts, and seeds. Including a variety of protein sources in the diet ensures that all essential amino acids are consumed, supporting optimal health.

Hydration is crucial during the third trimester to support the increased blood volume, amniotic fluid levels, and overall bodily functions. Adequate water intake can help prevent common issues such as constipation and urinary tract infections. Pregnant women should aim to drink at least 8-10 cups of water daily, and more if they are physically active or live in hot climates. Including hydrating foods like cucumbers, watermelon, and oranges in the diet can also contribute to overall hydration.

Fiber is important for digestive health, especially as the growing uterus can slow down the digestive system. Consuming plenty of fruits, vegetables, whole grains, and legumes can help maintain regular bowel movements and prevent constipation. Foods such as oats, berries, apples, and beans are rich in fiber and can be easily incorporated into meals and snacks.

Healthy fats are essential for energy, hormone production, and brain health. Sources of healthy fats include avocados, nuts, seeds, olive oil, and fatty fish like salmon. These fats can be included in meals and snacks to provide sustained energy and support overall health.

By focusing on these nutritional strategies, expectant mothers can ensure they have the energy, strength, and necessary nutrients for a healthy pregnancy, smooth delivery, and effective postpartum recovery.

Meal Planning and Snack Ideas
Staying nourished and maintaining energy levels during the third trimester can be managed with effective meal planning and incorporating nutritious snacks. Here are some practical meal and snack ideas that ensure a balanced intake of essential nutrients to support both mother and baby.

For breakfast, consider starting the day with a bowl of oatmeal topped with fresh berries, chia seeds, and a drizzle of honey. This meal provides a good balance of complex carbohydrates, fiber, antioxidants, and omega-3 fatty acids. Another option could be an avocado toast with whole-grain bread, a poached egg, and a sprinkle of pumpkin seeds, offering healthy fats, protein, and important vitamins and minerals.

Lunch should include a variety of food groups to ensure a balanced intake of nutrients. A quinoa salad with mixed greens, cherry tomatoes, cucumbers, feta cheese, and a lemon vinaigrette is both nutritious and satisfying. Alternatively, a turkey and avocado wrap with whole-grain tortillas, baby spinach, and a side of carrot sticks can provide a balanced meal rich in protein, fiber, and healthy fats.

For dinner, aim to include lean proteins, whole grains, and plenty of vegetables. Baked chicken with roasted sweet potatoes and steamed broccoli offers a well-rounded meal rich in vitamins, minerals, and protein. Another option could be a stir-fry with shrimp, bell peppers, snap peas, and brown rice, providing a colorful and nutrient-dense meal.

Snacks are an essential part of maintaining energy levels and preventing overeating at main meals. Healthy snack ideas include Greek yogurt with a handful of granola and sliced almonds, which offer protein, calcium, and healthy fats. Apple slices with peanut butter provide a satisfying combination of fiber and protein. A small bowl of mixed nuts can be a convenient and nutrient-dense option, offering healthy fats, protein, and important minerals like magnesium and zinc.

Smoothies can also be a great snack or meal option, especially when packed with nutrient-dense ingredients. A smoothie made with spinach, banana, almond milk, chia seeds, and a scoop of protein powder can provide a quick and nutritious boost.

Incorporating a variety of foods and maintaining a balanced diet through practical meal planning can help meet the nutritional needs of the third trimester. By focusing on whole foods and nutrient-dense options, expectant mothers can ensure they are providing the best possible nutrition for themselves and their growing babies, supporting a healthy pregnancy and preparing for the demands of labor and postpartum recovery.

Chapter 6

Mindful Weight Management During Pregnancy

Embarking on the journey of motherhood is a beautiful phase, filled with anticipation, joy, and a series of changes, both physical and emotional. One of the most significant aspects of this journey is managing weight during pregnancy, a crucial component of prenatal self-care. Weight management during pregnancy is not about adhering to strict diet plans or vigorous exercise regimes; rather, it's about nourishing your body and your baby with the right nutrients and maintaining a healthy balance.

The process of weight management during pregnancy involves understanding healthy weight gain, adopting mindful eating strategies, incorporating nutrient-dense foods into your diet, staying active safely, and creating personalized weight gain plans with the support of healthcare professionals. This chapter, "Mindful Weight Management During Pregnancy," will guide you through these essential aspects.

Healthy weight gain during pregnancy is vital for the well-being of both the mother and the developing baby. It supports the baby's growth and development while preparing the mother's body for labor and breastfeeding. The amount of weight gain recommended during pregnancy varies based on factors such as pre-pregnancy weight and body mass index (BMI). Generally, women with a normal BMI (18.5-24.9) are advised to gain between 25-35 pounds, while those underweight should aim for a gain of 28-40 pounds, and those overweight should target 15-25 pounds.

Mindful eating is a powerful tool for managing weight during pregnancy. It involves paying full attention to the experience of eating and listening to your body's hunger and fullness cues. This practice not only helps in maintaining a healthy weight but also fosters a positive relationship with food. Incorporating nutrient-dense foods into your diet is essential for healthy weight gain during pregnancy. These foods provide essential nutrients without excessive calories, ensuring that both you and your baby receive the necessary vitamins and minerals.

Physical activity during pregnancy is beneficial for both the mother and the baby. It helps manage weight, reduces the risk of gestational diabetes, improves mood, and promotes better sleep. However, it's important to choose exercises that are safe and appropriate for each stage of pregnancy. Every pregnancy is unique, and it's important to create a personalized weight gain plan in collaboration with your healthcare provider. This plan should consider your pre-pregnancy weight, BMI, and any existing health conditions to set realistic and healthy weight gain goals.

By approaching weight management mindfully, you can ensure that both you and your baby receive the best care possible, setting the foundation for a healthy pregnancy and beyond. Let's delve into the essential aspects of mindful weight management during this remarkable journey.

Understanding Healthy Weight Gain

Healthy weight gain during pregnancy is a cornerstone of prenatal care. It plays a critical role in ensuring both maternal and fetal health, influencing the pregnancy's outcome and the baby's development. The goal is not to simply add pounds but to foster a gradual, steady increase that supports the physiological changes of pregnancy.

During pregnancy, weight gain is distributed in various ways. This includes the baby's weight, the placenta, amniotic fluid, breast tissue, increased blood supply, fat stores, and the enlargement of the uterus. Each of these components is essential for a healthy pregnancy and delivery. Understanding this distribution helps in appreciating the importance of healthy weight gain.

The Institute of Medicine provides guidelines for weight gain during pregnancy based on pre-pregnancy BMI. For women with a normal BMI (18.5-24.9), the recommended gain is between 25-35 pounds. Those who are underweight (BMI less than 18.5) should aim for 28-40 pounds. Overweight women (BMI 25-29.9) are advised to gain 15-25 pounds, while obese women (BMI 30 and above) should limit weight gain to 11-20 pounds. These guidelines help ensure that both mother and baby remain healthy throughout pregnancy.

Appropriate weight gain supports the baby's growth and development and helps reduce the risk of complications such as preterm birth, low birth weight, and developmental issues. It also prepares the mother's body for the demands of labor and breastfeeding. On the other hand, excessive weight gain can lead to several health concerns, including gestational diabetes, preeclampsia, and the need for a cesarean section. It can also increase the risk of postpartum weight retention and obesity.

Excessive weight gain can pose long-term health risks for both mother and child. Mothers who gain too much weight during pregnancy are more likely to struggle with weight loss postpartum, increasing their risk of obesity and related conditions such as type 2 diabetes and cardiovascular disease. For the baby, excessive maternal weight gain can lead to a higher risk of childhood obesity, metabolic syndrome, and other health issues.

Monitoring weight gain is crucial, but it's equally important to focus on the quality of the diet and overall lifestyle. This involves eating a balanced diet rich in essential nutrients, staying physically active, and maintaining regular prenatal check-ups to monitor progress and make necessary adjustments. A holistic approach ensures that weight gain supports both the mother's and the baby's health without leading to unnecessary complications.

In summary, understanding healthy weight gain during pregnancy involves recognizing its importance, following recommended guidelines, and focusing on overall health rather than just the numbers on the scale. By doing so, expectant mothers can ensure they are providing the best possible environment for their baby's growth and development, while also taking care of their own health.

Mindful Eating Strategies

Mindful eating is a practice that encourages a healthier relationship with food by focusing on the present moment and acknowledging the sensory experience of eating. For pregnant women, this approach can be particularly beneficial in managing weight gain, reducing stress, and ensuring optimal nutrition for both mother and baby.

One of the core principles of mindful eating is paying attention to hunger and fullness cues. During pregnancy, your body's needs change, and it's important to listen to those changes. Before eating, take a moment to assess your hunger level. Are you physically hungry, or are you experiencing emotional hunger triggered by stress, boredom, or other emotions? Understanding the difference can help prevent overeating and emotional eating.

To practice mindful eating, start by setting aside dedicated time for meals. Avoid distractions such as phones, television, or work while eating. Focus on the act of eating itself—notice the colors, textures, and flavors of your food. Chew slowly and thoroughly, savoring each bite. This not only enhances the eating experience but also allows your body to signal when it is full, helping to prevent overeating.

Cravings are common during pregnancy, and mindful eating can help manage them without leading to excessive weight gain. When a craving strikes, pause and consider whether it is driven by genuine hunger or an emotional response. If it's a craving for something specific, find a healthier alternative that still satisfies your taste. For instance, if you crave something sweet, opt for a piece of fruit or a small serving of yogurt with honey.

Another aspect of mindful eating is planning and preparing balanced meals. Focus on including a variety of nutrient-dense foods that provide essential vitamins and minerals for you and your baby. Lean proteins, whole grains, fruits, vegetables, and healthy fats should form the basis of your diet. Planning meals ahead of time can help you make healthier choices and avoid last-minute, less nutritious options.

It's also important to stay hydrated. Sometimes, thirst can be mistaken for hunger, leading to unnecessary snacking. Drinking plenty of water throughout the day helps maintain hydration, supports digestion, and can prevent overeating. Aim for at least eight glasses of water daily, more if you are physically active or live in a hot climate.

Mindful eating is not about strict rules or deprivation. It's about creating a positive, balanced relationship with food. Allow yourself to enjoy your favorite treats in moderation. Depriving yourself can lead to feelings of frustration and may trigger binge eating. Instead, practice portion control and savor those indulgent moments without guilt.

Finally, consider keeping a food journal to track your eating habits. This can help identify patterns and triggers for emotional eating and provide insight into how well you are meeting your nutritional needs. Share this journal with your healthcare provider during prenatal visits to receive personalized advice and support.

Mindful eating strategies can significantly contribute to healthy weight management during pregnancy. By paying attention to hunger and fullness cues, managing cravings thoughtfully, and focusing on balanced, nutrient-dense meals, expectant mothers can nourish their bodies and their babies effectively. This approach promotes a healthier relationship with food and supports overall well-being during this transformative time.

Nutrient-Dense Foods for Weight Management

Maintaining a diet rich in nutrient-dense foods is essential for healthy weight management during pregnancy. Nutrient-dense foods provide the vitamins, minerals, and other essential nutrients needed for the baby's development and the mother's health, without adding excessive calories.

Lean proteins are a crucial part of a pregnancy diet. They are the building blocks of your baby's cells and tissues, supporting growth and development. Sources of lean protein include chicken, turkey, fish, eggs, beans, lentils, and tofu. Incorporating a source of protein in every meal helps keep you feeling full and supports stable energy levels throughout the day.

Whole grains are another important component of a balanced pregnancy diet. They are rich in complex carbohydrates, which provide a steady source of energy, and fiber, which aids digestion and helps prevent constipation—a common issue during pregnancy. Examples of whole grains include brown rice, quinoa, oats, whole wheat bread, and barley. These grains also supply important nutrients like B vitamins, iron, and magnesium.

Fruits and vegetables should make up a significant portion of your diet. They are low in calories but high in essential vitamins, minerals, and fiber. Aim to fill half your plate with fruits and vegetables at each meal. Dark leafy greens like spinach and kale are particularly beneficial due to their high content of folate, a critical nutrient for preventing neural tube defects in the developing baby. Other nutrient-dense vegetables include broccoli, carrots, bell peppers, and sweet potatoes.

Fruits like berries, apples, bananas, and oranges provide vital nutrients and antioxidants. They can also satisfy sweet cravings in a healthy way. Opt for fresh, frozen, or canned fruits without added sugars. Remember to wash all fruits and vegetables thoroughly to reduce the risk of exposure to harmful bacteria or pesticides.

Healthy fats are also important for fetal development, particularly for brain and eye health. Sources of healthy fats include avocados, nuts, seeds, olive oil, and fatty fish like salmon and sardines. Omega-3 fatty acids, found in fatty fish and flaxseeds, are especially beneficial for brain development. Including a source of healthy fat in each meal can help you feel satisfied and support your baby's growth.

Dairy products or fortified plant-based alternatives provide calcium, which is essential for the development of your baby's bones and teeth. Dairy products also supply protein and vitamin D. If you are lactose intolerant or prefer non-dairy options, choose fortified plant-based milks like almond, soy, or oat milk. Yogurt and cheese are also excellent sources of calcium and can be included in your diet as snacks or part of meals.

Hydration is another critical aspect of nutrition during pregnancy. Water supports many bodily functions, including digestion and nutrient absorption. It also helps maintain amniotic fluid levels, which are essential for the baby's protection and development. Aim to drink at least eight glasses of water a day, and more if you are physically active. Herbal teas and water-rich foods like fruits and vegetables can also contribute to your daily hydration needs.

It's important to avoid empty-calorie foods that provide little nutritional value but can contribute to excessive weight gain. These include sugary snacks, sodas, and processed foods high in unhealthy fats and sugars. While occasional indulgences are fine, focusing on nutrient-dense choices will benefit both you and your baby in the long run.

Incorporating nutrient-dense foods into your pregnancy diet is key to managing healthy weight gain. Lean proteins, whole grains, fruits, vegetables, healthy fats, and dairy products provide the essential nutrients needed for your baby's development and your well-being. By prioritizing these foods and staying hydrated, you can support a healthy pregnancy and set the foundation for lifelong health.

Staying Active During Pregnancy

Staying active during pregnancy is not only safe for most women but also highly beneficial. Regular physical activity helps manage weight, reduces the risk of gestational diabetes and preeclampsia, improves mood, and promotes better sleep. Additionally, it can help prepare your body for labor and recovery postpartum.

Before starting or continuing an exercise routine during pregnancy, it's important to consult with your healthcare provider. They can offer personalized advice based on your health and pregnancy status, ensuring that you engage in safe and appropriate activities.

For most pregnant women, the goal is to maintain a moderate level of physical activity, aiming for about 150 minutes of moderate-intensity exercise per week. This can be broken down into 30-minute sessions on most days of the week. Here are some safe and effective exercises for each trimester:

First Trimester:
During the first trimester, many women experience fatigue and morning sickness, which can make it challenging to stay active. However, gentle exercises such as walking, swimming, and prenatal yoga can be beneficial. Walking is a great way to stay active without putting too much strain on your body. Swimming and water aerobics are also excellent options, as they provide a full-body workout while minimizing stress on the joints.

Second Trimester:
The second trimester is often considered the most comfortable period for exercise, as many women experience increased energy levels and a reduction in morning sickness. At this stage, you can continue with walking, swimming, and prenatal yoga, and consider adding light strength training to your routine. Strength training helps maintain muscle tone and support your changing body. Focus on exercises that strengthen the back, abdomen, and pelvic floor muscles. Always use light weights and avoid exercises that involve lying flat on your back after the first trimester.

Third Trimester:

As your pregnancy progresses into the third trimester, your center of gravity shifts, and you may experience increased discomfort. Low-impact exercises like walking, swimming, and prenatal yoga remain good choices. Pelvic floor exercises, such as Kegels, are particularly important during this stage, as they help prepare the body for labor and support recovery postpartum. Gentle stretching and relaxation exercises can also help alleviate discomfort and improve flexibility.

Regardless of the trimester, it's important to listen to your body and avoid overexertion. Signs that you should stop exercising and consult your healthcare provider include dizziness, shortness of breath, chest pain, headache, uterine contractions, vaginal bleeding, or fluid leakage. Staying hydrated and avoiding exercise in extreme heat are also crucial to ensure safety.

Incorporating more movement into your daily routine can also be beneficial. Simple activities like taking the stairs instead of the elevator, walking to nearby errands, or engaging in light household chores can help you stay active without a structured exercise regimen. Prenatal exercise classes, either in-person or online, can provide guidance and motivation while ensuring that you are performing safe and effective exercises.

Physical activity during pregnancy offers numerous benefits beyond weight management. It helps reduce stress, improve sleep quality, and boost overall mood. Exercise can also alleviate common pregnancy discomforts such as back pain, constipation, and swelling. Moreover, staying active can enhance your stamina and endurance, which can be beneficial during labor and delivery.

Staying active during pregnancy is essential for both physical and mental well-being. By choosing safe and appropriate exercises for each trimester, you can manage weight, improve mood, and prepare your body for the demands of labor and postpartum recovery. Always consult with your healthcare provider before starting any exercise program and listen to your body to ensure a safe and healthy pregnancy.

Personalized Weight Gain Plans and Self-Care

Every pregnancy is unique, and so are the needs and experiences of each expectant mother. Creating a personalized weight gain plan in collaboration with your healthcare provider is crucial to ensure that you and your baby receive the best possible care. This plan should take into account your pre-pregnancy weight, body mass index (BMI), any existing health conditions, and your overall lifestyle.

To start, discuss your weight gain goals with your healthcare provider during your initial prenatal visit. They can help determine the appropriate weight gain range based on your individual circumstances. Regular follow-up appointments allow for monitoring your progress and making adjustments as needed. Your healthcare provider can offer personalized advice on diet, exercise, and any necessary supplements to support your health and your baby's development.

A personalized weight gain plan focuses not just on the amount of weight gained but also on the quality of that gain. Emphasizing a balanced diet rich in nutrient-dense foods is essential. Lean proteins, whole grains, fruits, vegetables, healthy fats, and dairy products should form the foundation of your diet. Your healthcare provider can help identify any specific nutritional needs or deficiencies and recommend appropriate adjustments or supplements.

Self-care is an integral part of managing weight and maintaining overall well-being during pregnancy. Practicing self-compassion and maintaining a positive body image can significantly impact your mental and emotional health. Pregnancy brings about many physical changes, and it's important to embrace these changes with kindness and understanding. Remind yourself that these changes are part of the beautiful process of creating new life.

Incorporating self-care practices into your daily routine can help manage stress and promote a positive mindset. This can include activities such as prenatal yoga, meditation, deep breathing exercises, or simply taking time each day to relax and unwind. Engaging in hobbies and activities that bring you joy and fulfillment is also important for maintaining emotional well-being.

Maintaining a positive body image during pregnancy can be challenging, especially with societal pressures and comparisons. Surround yourself with supportive people who uplift and encourage you. Avoid negative self-talk and focus on the amazing things your body is doing. Celebrate the milestones of your pregnancy and recognize the strength and resilience of your body.

Another important aspect of self-care is ensuring adequate rest and sleep. Pregnancy can be physically demanding, and getting enough rest is crucial for both you and your baby. Aim for 7-9 hours of sleep each night and take naps if needed. Establishing a relaxing bedtime routine can help improve sleep quality.

Seeking support from others can also be beneficial. Joining a prenatal support group or attending childbirth classes can provide a sense of community and shared experience. These groups offer a space to discuss concerns, share advice, and receive emotional support from others who are going through similar experiences.

Lastly, it's important to recognize that every pregnancy journey is different. What works for one person may not work for another. Be open to adjusting your plan as needed and communicate regularly with your healthcare provider. They can help navigate any challenges and provide guidance tailored to your specific needs.

Creating a personalized weight gain plan and prioritizing self-care are essential components of a healthy pregnancy. Collaborate with your healthcare provider to set realistic and healthy goals, focus on a balanced and nutrient-dense diet, and incorporate self-care practices to support your mental and emotional well-being. Embrace the changes your body goes through and maintain a positive mindset throughout this remarkable journey. By doing so, you can ensure that both you and your baby receive the best care possible, setting the foundation for a healthy and fulfilling pregnancy.

Chapter 7

Dietary Solutions for Common Pregnancy Symptoms and Conditions

As someone who's experienced the joys and challenges of pregnancy firsthand, I understand that it can be quite an overwhelming journey. Despite the discomforts we might face, one thing remains certain - your nutrition matters. This chapter of "Prenatal Nutrition: A Self-Care Approach to Nourishing Your Body and Baby," we're going to explore how dietary choices can significantly ease common pregnancy symptoms.

We'll go into managing morning sickness with strategic food choices and snacking habits. We'll discuss how your diet can help reduce heartburn and indigestion, two discomforting realities many expectant mothers face. Another major aspect we will explore is that of gestational diabetes; you would be amazed at how much of a role your diet plays in managing this condition.

We'll also talk about other common complaints during pregnancy, such as constipation, bloating, and fatigue, and how they can all be alleviated with the right nutrition strategies. And, of course, we will discuss meal planning and smart snacking for symptom relief – a practical guide that you can easily incorporate into your daily routines.

Throughout this chapter, I'll share personal experiences, tips, and stories that I hope will help you through your pregnancy journey. Remember, self-care begins with good nutrition. Every bite we consume can make a world of difference to our bodies and to our babies.

Morning Sickness: Foods to Ease the Discomfort

I remember my first trimester - the morning sickness was ruthless. But let me share how foods like ginger-infused teas and crackers before rising helped me deal with nausea. When the waves of nausea hit, I found that small, frequent meals were my best friend. Eating a couple of plain crackers or dry toast before getting out of bed in the morning helped settle my stomach. Ginger, in various forms, became a staple - ginger tea, ginger ale, and even ginger candies.

Cold foods sometimes felt more palatable than hot ones, and munching on chilled fruits like watermelon and grapes provided not only relief but also hydration. Bananas were another go-to, as they are gentle on the stomach and provide essential nutrients. High-protein snacks such as nuts and seeds also helped stabilize my blood sugar levels, reducing the intensity of nausea.

Staying hydrated was crucial, but plain water often felt unappealing. Sipping on flavored water, herbal teas, or even sucking on ice chips was more manageable. Peppermint tea was another soothing option that calmed my stomach.

I learned to avoid foods and smells that triggered nausea. For me, greasy or fried foods and strong odors were the main culprits. Instead, I opted for bland, easy-to-digest foods like rice, applesauce, and plain potatoes. Keeping a food diary to track what worked and what didn't was incredibly helpful in navigating this period.

Incorporating these strategies and foods into my daily routine made a significant difference. I found that focusing on nutrient-dense snacks and staying hydrated were key in managing morning sickness. Listening to my body and being gentle with myself also helped me cope better during those challenging first few months.

Food Choices to Reduce Heartburn and Indigestion

Heartburn and indigestion seemed to become frequent uninvited guests during my pregnancy. I quickly realized that certain foods and habits could either trigger or alleviate these discomforts. For instance, spicy, fatty, and acidic foods were major triggers for me. Dishes with a lot of spices, citrus fruits, tomatoes, and even chocolate seemed to worsen the heartburn. So, I had to adjust my diet accordingly.

I began to incorporate more alkaline foods, such as bananas, melons, and cucumbers, which are known to neutralize stomach acid. Lean proteins like grilled chicken and fish, along with whole grains like oatmeal and brown rice, also became staples in my diet. These foods are not only nutritious but also gentle on the digestive system.

Eating smaller, more frequent meals instead of three large ones helped manage indigestion. Overeating can exacerbate heartburn, so I focused on portion control and mindfulness while eating. I made sure to chew my food thoroughly and avoid lying down immediately after meals. Propping myself up with pillows when resting or sleeping also helped prevent acid reflux.

Dairy products, particularly milk and yogurt, provided soothing relief. A glass of milk or a serving of yogurt helped coat my stomach and reduce the burning sensation. However, I was mindful of dairy intake, as too much could lead to other digestive issues.

Staying hydrated was essential, but I avoided drinking large amounts of water during meals, which can dilute stomach acids and impair digestion. Instead, I sipped water throughout the day and included herbal teas, like chamomile, which helped with digestion and provided a calming effect.

By making these dietary adjustments and adopting mindful eating practices, I managed to significantly reduce the frequency and severity of heartburn and indigestion. Each expectant mother is different, so finding what works best for you might take some trial and error, but the relief is well worth the effort.

Managing Gestational Diabetes through Diet

Upon being diagnosed with gestational diabetes during my second pregnancy, I had to revisit my plate. It isn't as terrifying as it sounds. Let me guide you through my diet adjustments. Managing gestational diabetes revolves around keeping blood sugar levels stable, which means paying close attention to carbohydrate intake and focusing on balanced meals.

One of the first changes I made was incorporating complex carbohydrates instead of simple ones. Whole grains like quinoa, brown rice, and whole wheat bread replaced white bread, rice, and pasta. These complex carbs are digested more slowly, leading to more stable blood sugar levels.

I also ensured that each meal contained a good balance of protein, healthy fats, and fiber. Proteins like lean meats, eggs, and beans, along with healthy fats from avocados, nuts, and olive oil, helped maintain steady blood sugar levels. Fiber-rich foods, such as vegetables, fruits, and legumes, were also crucial as they slow the absorption of sugar.

Meal timing became another important aspect. Eating smaller, more frequent meals every 2-3 hours helped prevent blood sugar spikes and dips. Breakfast was particularly important to start the day right. I often had a protein-rich smoothie with spinach, berries, and a scoop of protein powder, or a bowl of oatmeal with nuts and seeds.

Snacking wisely was another strategy that helped manage my blood sugar. I found that pairing a carbohydrate with a protein or fat made a significant difference. For example, an apple with a handful of almonds, or whole-grain crackers with cheese, provided sustained energy without causing spikes in blood sugar.

Foods high in sugar and refined carbohydrates were off the table. I avoided sweets, sugary drinks, and processed snacks. Instead, I satisfied my sweet tooth with fruits like berries, which have a lower glycemic index, and used natural sweeteners like stevia in moderation.

Staying hydrated and keeping active also played vital roles in managing gestational diabetes. Regular walks and prenatal exercises helped improve insulin sensitivity, making it easier to control blood sugar levels.

By making these dietary adjustments and staying committed to a balanced eating plan, I was able to manage my gestational diabetes effectively. It required discipline and careful planning, but the health benefits for both me and my baby were worth the effort.

Bottle gourd and spinach were my go-to foods to combat constipation, while yogurt and bananas helped me with bloating. Does fatigue bog you down? I have some tips for that too. During pregnancy, managing common complaints through nutrition can make a significant difference in comfort and well-being.

For constipation, increasing fiber intake was key. Foods like prunes, whole grains, and leafy greens were incredibly helpful. Prunes, either eaten whole or as juice, are natural laxatives that kept things moving. Whole grains, such as oatmeal, brown rice, and whole wheat bread, provided soluble fiber that softened stools. Spinach and other leafy greens added bulk and aided digestion. Staying hydrated by drinking plenty of water also played a crucial role in preventing constipation.

Bloating can be quite uncomfortable, and I found that certain foods and habits helped alleviate this. Yogurt, with its probiotics, aided digestion and reduced bloating. Bananas, rich in potassium, helped balance sodium levels and reduced water retention. Avoiding carbonated drinks and chewing gum, which introduce excess air into the digestive system, also minimized bloating.

Fatigue is another common issue during pregnancy, and addressing it through diet can be effective. Iron-rich foods like lean meats, beans, and fortified cereals helped combat anemia-related fatigue. Vitamin C-rich foods, such as oranges and strawberries, enhanced iron absorption. Including a mix of complex carbs and proteins in meals provided sustained energy. For instance, a lunch of grilled chicken with quinoa and steamed vegetables kept me energized throughout the day.

Hydration is essential for overall health, and during pregnancy, it becomes even more important. Drinking at least eight glasses of water a day kept me hydrated and helped with digestion, circulation, and the absorption of nutrients. Herbal teas and water-rich foods like cucumbers and watermelon also contributed to my daily hydration needs.

Managing cravings was another aspect I had to navigate. Cravings can sometimes lead to unhealthy choices, but I found ways to satisfy them healthily. Craving sweets? A bowl of mixed berries with a dollop of Greek yogurt did the trick. Craving something salty? Air-popped popcorn seasoned with herbs was a great alternative to chips. Keeping healthy snacks like nuts, seeds, and fruits readily available helped me make better choices.

By focusing on these nutrition strategies, I was able to manage common pregnancy complaints effectively. It took some planning and discipline, but the improvement in comfort and overall well-being was worth it. Remember, every small dietary adjustment can make a big difference in how you feel during pregnancy.

Meal Planning and Snacking for Symptom Relief

Planning meals and snacks isn't just about filling our stomachs - it's more strategic than that during pregnancy. Here are some sample meal plans and snack ideas that worked wonders in easing my symptoms. Incorporating symptom-easing foods into a regular diet can be simple and delicious.

For breakfast, I often started my day with a smoothie bowl. Blending spinach, frozen berries, a banana, and a scoop of protein powder created a nutrient-packed meal. Topping it with chia seeds and nuts added fiber and healthy fats. Another favorite was oatmeal topped with fresh fruits and a drizzle of honey.

Lunches were light yet satisfying. A quinoa salad with mixed greens, cherry tomatoes, cucumbers, and grilled chicken was a staple. I dressed it with a simple olive oil and lemon vinaigrette. Another option was a whole-grain wrap filled with hummus, sliced veggies, and lean turkey. These meals were easy to prepare and packed with nutrients.

Dinners focused on balance and variety. A typical dinner included a piece of grilled salmon, a side of roasted sweet potatoes, and steamed broccoli. This combination provided protein, healthy fats, and fiber. Another favorite was a stir-fry with tofu, mixed vegetables, and brown rice. Adding ginger and garlic not only enhanced the flavor but also offered additional health benefits.

Snacking smartly throughout the day helped manage symptoms and maintain energy levels. Greek yogurt with a handful of berries and a sprinkle of granola was a frequent choice. A small bowl of trail mix, made with nuts, seeds, and dried fruits, provided a good mix of protein and fiber. Veggie sticks with hummus or guacamole were also great for satisfying hunger between meals.

Incorporating symptom-easing foods into my diet required a bit of planning, but it soon became second nature. I focused on whole, unprocessed foods and included a variety of fruits, vegetables, lean proteins, and whole grains in every meal. Keeping a well-stocked pantry with healthy options made it easier to stick to my plan.

Batch cooking and meal prepping on weekends saved time and reduced stress during the week. I would prepare large batches of quinoa, roast a variety of vegetables, and grill several portions of chicken or fish. Storing these in the fridge allowed me to mix and match components for quick and nutritious meals.

By following these meal planning and snacking strategies, I found that managing pregnancy symptoms became much more manageable. The right nutrition not only supported my health but also eased the discomforts of pregnancy, making the journey smoother and more enjoyable.

This chapter is filled with not just clinical information but also personal experiences, tips, and stories that I hope will help you through your pregnancy journey. Remember, self-care begins with good nutrition. Every bite we consume can make a world of difference to our bodies and to our babies.

Chapter 8

Superfoods for Pregnancy: Boosting Health for Mother and Baby

As a mother-to-be, ensuring that I was nourishing myself and my growing baby with the right foods quickly became one of my top priorities. I soon realized that while eating a balanced diet is crucial, incorporating superfoods can provide an extra boost. Superfoods are nutrient-rich foods that offer significant health benefits. During pregnancy, these foods can support both maternal health and fetal development in remarkable ways.

In this chapter, "Superfoods for Pregnancy: Boosting Health for Mother and Baby," we will explore a range of superfoods that can make a significant difference in your pregnancy journey. From leafy greens bursting with essential minerals to antioxidant-rich berries, omega-3 packed fish, nutritious nuts and seeds, calcium-rich dairy, carotenoid-packed sweet potatoes, wholesome fermented foods, fiber-filled whole grains, and anti-inflammatory herbs and spices, each of these superfoods can play a vital role in ensuring both you and your baby are healthy and strong.

I'll share personal experiences, tips, and practical advice on how to incorporate these powerful nutrition powerhouses into your daily meals. Whether it's through simple recipes, snack ideas, or easy meal additions, this guide aims to make your journey through pregnancy a nourishing and enjoyable experience. Remember, self-care begins with what you eat, and every bite can make a significant impact on your health and your baby's development.

Leafy Greens

When I first learned about the importance of leafy greens during pregnancy, I was amazed at how much these humble vegetables could offer. Spinach, kale, collard greens, and Swiss chard quickly became staples in my diet, providing a wealth of nutrients crucial for both my health and my baby's development.

Leafy greens are packed with folate, a vital B-vitamin that supports neural tube development and helps prevent birth defects of the brain and spine. They are also rich in iron, which is essential for preventing anemia, a common concern during pregnancy. Additionally, these greens are loaded with calcium, supporting bone health for both mother and baby, and vitamins A and C, which boost the immune system and aid in skin health.

I found that incorporating leafy greens into my diet was easier than I initially thought. Smoothies became my go-to breakfast, where I could blend a handful of spinach or kale with fruits like bananas and berries for a nutrient-dense start to the day. Salads with mixed greens, topped with a variety of colorful vegetables, nuts, and seeds, made for a refreshing and nutritious lunch or dinner.

Cooking leafy greens is also a great way to include them in your diet. Sautéing spinach or Swiss chard with a bit of garlic and olive oil, or adding them to soups and stews, can make a comforting and healthful meal. Kale chips, baked with a light seasoning of sea salt, offer a crunchy and satisfying snack.

One of my favorite ways to enjoy leafy greens is in a frittata. Beaten eggs mixed with sautéed spinach, kale, onions, and a bit of cheese, then baked until golden, make for a delicious and nutritious breakfast or brunch option.

By making leafy greens a regular part of my meals, I felt more energized and confident that I was providing my baby with essential nutrients. It's incredible how these versatile vegetables can be so beneficial and easy to include in your daily diet.

Berries

Berries quickly became a favorite part of my diet during pregnancy. Strawberries, blueberries, raspberries, and blackberries are not only delicious but also pack a powerful punch of nutrients that are incredibly beneficial for both mother and baby.

These colorful fruits are rich in antioxidants, which help protect the body from oxidative stress and support the immune system. Berries are also a fantastic source of vitamin C, which is crucial for the growth and repair of tissues and aids in the absorption of iron from other foods. Additionally, they provide a good amount of fiber, helping to maintain healthy digestion and prevent constipation, a common issue during pregnancy.

I found that berries were one of the easiest superfoods to incorporate into my diet. They make a perfect snack on their own, but I also loved adding them to my breakfast. A bowl of oatmeal topped with a mix of fresh berries and a drizzle of honey became a staple morning meal. Greek yogurt with a handful of berries and a sprinkle of granola also made for a quick and nutritious start to the day.

Smoothies were another favorite way to enjoy berries. Blending a mix of strawberries, blueberries, a banana, and a splash of almond milk created a refreshing and nutrient-packed drink that I could enjoy on the go. Sometimes, I would add a handful of spinach to my berry smoothies for an extra boost of vitamins and minerals without altering the delicious flavor.

For a sweet treat, I enjoyed making berry parfaits. Layering Greek yogurt, mixed berries, and a bit of granola in a glass created a beautiful and satisfying dessert that was both healthy and indulgent. Berries also made a great addition to salads, adding a pop of color and natural sweetness that complemented leafy greens and other vegetables perfectly.

Including berries in my diet not only provided essential nutrients but also made my meals more enjoyable and flavorful. Their versatility and health benefits make them an excellent choice for expectant mothers looking to boost their nutrition in a delicious way.

Fatty Fish

Fatty fish like salmon, mackerel, and sardines were some of the most beneficial additions to my diet during pregnancy. These fish are rich in omega-3 fatty acids, particularly DHA and EPA, which are crucial for the development of the baby's brain and eyes. Omega-3s also support maternal heart health and can reduce the risk of preterm birth.

One of the key nutrients in fatty fish is vitamin D, which helps with calcium absorption and bone health. This is especially important during pregnancy as the baby's bones develop. Additionally, fatty fish are a great source of high-quality protein, which is essential for the growth and repair of tissues.

Incorporating fatty fish into my diet was both enjoyable and rewarding. I often grilled or baked salmon with a simple seasoning of lemon, herbs, and olive oil. Pairing it with a side of steamed vegetables and quinoa made for a well-balanced and nutritious meal. For a quick and easy lunch, I loved making salmon salads with mixed greens, avocado, and a light vinaigrette.

Sardines, although not everyone's favorite, are incredibly nutrient-dense and can be enjoyed in various ways. I found that adding them to a Mediterranean-style salad with tomatoes, cucumbers, olives, and feta cheese was a tasty and satisfying option. Sardines on whole-grain toast with a squeeze of lemon juice and a sprinkle of black pepper also made for a nutritious snack.

Fish tacos were another delightful way to include fatty fish in my meals. Grilling pieces of seasoned mackerel and serving them in whole-grain tortillas with a fresh slaw and avocado was a fun and delicious dinner option that my whole family enjoyed.

One thing to keep in mind is to choose low-mercury fish and limit intake to recommended levels. The FDA advises pregnant women to consume 2-3 servings (8-12 ounces) of low-mercury fish per week to maximize benefits while minimizing risks.

By including fatty fish in my diet, I felt confident that I was supporting my baby's development and my own health. The variety of ways to prepare and enjoy these fish made it easy to incorporate them into my weekly meal plans.

Nuts and Seeds
Nuts and seeds became a go-to snack during my pregnancy. Almonds, walnuts, chia seeds, and flaxseeds are just a few of the nutrient-dense options that provided essential vitamins and minerals. These tiny powerhouses are packed with healthy fats, protein, fiber, and a range of vitamins and minerals that support both maternal health and fetal development.

Almonds, for instance, are rich in vitamin E, which is important for skin health and acts as an antioxidant. They also provide magnesium, which helps with muscle relaxation and can prevent cramps, a common issue during pregnancy. Walnuts are an excellent source of omega-3 fatty acids, particularly ALA, which supports brain health. Chia seeds and flaxseeds are also high in omega-3s, as well as fiber, which aids in digestion and helps prevent constipation.

One of my favorite ways to enjoy nuts and seeds was by adding them to my morning oatmeal or yogurt. A handful of mixed nuts and a sprinkle of chia seeds added a satisfying crunch and boosted the nutritional value of my meals. I also loved making homemade trail mix with almonds, walnuts, dried cranberries, and dark chocolate chips for a convenient and healthy snack.

Nut butters, such as almond or peanut butter, were another staple in my diet. Spreading a bit of almond butter on whole-grain toast or apple slices made for a delicious and nutrient-rich snack. I also enjoyed adding a spoonful of nut butter to smoothies for added creaminess and nutrition.

Seeds, particularly chia and flax seeds, were easy to incorporate into various dishes. I often added a tablespoon of chia seeds to my smoothies or yogurt, which helped keep me feeling full and provided a good dose of omega-3s and fiber. Flaxseeds, when ground, can be added to baked goods, oatmeal, or sprinkled over salads.

Nuts and seeds also made great additions to salads, providing a crunchy texture and a boost of nutrients. A spinach salad with walnuts, feta cheese, and a balsamic vinaigrette became one of my favorite lunch options.

Including nuts and seeds in my diet was an easy and tasty way to ensure I was getting a variety of essential nutrients. Their versatility and convenience made them a perfect snack and addition to meals, supporting both my health and my baby's development.

Dairy and Fortified Plant-Based Alternatives

Dairy products and fortified plant-based alternatives played a crucial role in my diet during pregnancy. They are excellent sources of calcium, vitamin D, protein, and other essential nutrients that support bone health and overall development.

Dairy products like milk, yogurt, and cheese are rich in calcium, which is vital for the development of the baby's bones and teeth. They also provide vitamin D, which helps with calcium absorption and supports immune function. Greek yogurt, in particular, became a favorite of mine due to its high protein content and creamy texture. It's also a good source of probiotics, which support digestive health.

For those who are lactose intolerant or prefer plant-based options, fortified plant-based milks such as almond, soy, and oat milk are great alternatives. These are often fortified with calcium, vitamin D, and other essential nutrients to match the nutritional profile of dairy milk. I found that switching between dairy and plant-based milks added variety to my diet and ensured I was getting the necessary nutrients.

One of my favorite breakfast options was a bowl of Greek yogurt topped with fresh berries, a drizzle of honey, and a sprinkle of granola. This not only provided a good dose of calcium and protein but also added a delicious crunch and sweetness to start my day. Smoothies made with fortified almond milk, a banana, and a handful of spinach also became a regular part of my morning routine.

Cheese, in moderation, was another enjoyable way to include dairy in my diet. Adding a bit of feta or cheddar to salads, or enjoying a slice of whole-grain bread with some cheese and a piece of fruit made for a satisfying snack

For plant-based alternatives, I loved making chia pudding with fortified almond milk. Mixing chia seeds with almond milk and letting it sit overnight in the fridge created a delicious and nutrient-packed pudding that I could enjoy for breakfast or as a snack.

Incorporating dairy and fortified plant-based alternatives into my diet was not only easy but also enjoyable. These foods provided essential nutrients that supported my health and my baby's development, making them an integral part of my pregnancy nutrition plan.

Sweet Potatoes and Carotenoid-Rich Foods
Sweet potatoes quickly became one of my favorite superfoods during pregnancy. These vibrant orange tubers are packed with beta-carotene, a type of carotenoid that the body converts into vitamin A. Vitamin A is essential for the development of the baby's eyes, skin, and immune system.

In addition to sweet potatoes, other carotenoid-rich foods like carrots, pumpkins, and butternut squash also provide a wealth of nutrients. These foods are high in antioxidants, which help protect the body from oxidative stress, and they support overall health during pregnancy.

One of the best things about sweet potatoes is their versatility. I loved baking them in the oven with a bit of olive oil, salt, and pepper for a simple and delicious side dish. Mashed sweet potatoes with a touch of cinnamon and a dollop of Greek yogurt made for a comforting and nutritious meal. Sweet potato fries, baked until crispy, were another favorite snack or side dish.

Carrots were easy to incorporate into my diet as well. I often added shredded carrots to salads, soups, and stir-fries for an extra boost of nutrients and a bit of sweetness. Roasting carrots with a drizzle of honey and a sprinkle of herbs created a delicious and colorful side dish.

Pumpkin and butternut squash were great for making soups and stews. A creamy pumpkin soup with a bit of ginger and coconut milk became a comforting and nutrient-rich meal during the colder months. Butternut squash roasted with sage and a bit of parmesan cheese was another favorite dish.

One of the most enjoyable ways to include carotenoid-rich foods in my diet was through smoothies. Blending cooked sweet potatoes or pumpkin with a banana, a handful of spinach, and a splash of almond milk created a creamy and nutrient-dense smoothie that I could enjoy for breakfast or as a snack.

By including sweet potatoes and other carotenoid-rich foods in my meals, I felt confident that I was providing my baby with essential nutrients while also enjoying delicious and satisfying dishes. Their vibrant colors and natural sweetness made them a delightful addition to my pregnancy diet.

Fermented Foods

Fermented foods were a surprising and beneficial addition to my diet during pregnancy. Foods like yogurt, kefir, sauerkraut, kimchi, and miso are rich in probiotics, which are beneficial bacteria that support gut health. A healthy gut microbiome is important for overall well-being and can help improve digestion, boost the immune system, and even influence mood.

Yogurt and kefir became staples in my daily routine. Greek yogurt, in particular, was not only high in protein but also provided a good amount of probiotics. I enjoyed it with fresh fruit and a drizzle of honey for breakfast or as a snack. Kefir, a fermented milk drink, was another great way to include probiotics in my diet. It has a tangy flavor and can be enjoyed on its own or blended into smoothies.

Sauerkraut and kimchi, fermented cabbage dishes, were delicious additions to my meals. I often added a spoonful of sauerkraut to my salads or as a side dish with grilled meats. Kimchi, with its spicy and tangy flavor, was a perfect complement to rice bowls and stir-fries. Both of these fermented vegetables provided probiotics and added a burst of flavor to my meals.

Miso, a fermented soybean paste, was another favorite. Miso soup, made with a simple broth, tofu, seaweed, and green onions, was a comforting and nutritious dish. I also used miso as a seasoning in marinades and dressings, adding a depth of flavor to my cooking.

Incorporating fermented foods into my diet not only supported my digestive health but also added a variety of flavors and textures to my meals. These foods were easy to include and made a noticeable difference in how I felt during my pregnancy. The probiotics helped maintain a healthy gut, which in turn supported my overall well-being and immune system.

Whole Grains
Whole grains were a crucial part of my diet during pregnancy, providing essential nutrients and sustained energy. Foods like quinoa, brown rice, oats, and whole wheat products are rich in fiber, B vitamins, iron, and magnesium, all of which are important for both maternal health and fetal development.

Quinoa, a complete protein containing all nine essential amino acids, became a staple in my meals. I enjoyed it as a base for salads, mixed with vegetables, beans, and a light dressing. Quinoa also made a great addition to soups and stews, adding both texture and nutrition. For breakfast, quinoa porridge with a bit of cinnamon, honey, and fresh fruit was a hearty and nutritious start to the day.

Brown rice was another favorite whole grain. It provided a good source of complex carbohydrates and fiber, helping to keep me full and energized throughout the day. I often paired brown rice with stir-fries, curries, or simply mixed it with steamed vegetables and a bit of soy sauce for a quick and easy meal.

Oats were a breakfast staple that I never got tired of. Overnight oats, made by soaking oats in milk or a plant-based alternative and adding fruits, nuts, and seeds, were a convenient and delicious way to start my morning. Warm oatmeal topped with berries, a dollop of Greek yogurt, and a sprinkle of chia seeds was another favorite breakfast option.

Whole wheat products, such as whole wheat bread, pasta, and tortillas, were easy to include in my diet and provided additional fiber and nutrients. Whole wheat toast with avocado and a poached egg made for a satisfying breakfast or snack. Whole wheat pasta with a variety of vegetables and a homemade tomato sauce was a comforting and nutritious dinner option.

By choosing whole grains over refined grains, I ensured that I was getting more fiber, vitamins, and minerals in my diet. These foods not only supported my digestive health but also provided sustained energy, which was especially important during pregnancy.

Herbs and Spices

Herbs and spices added flavor and a range of health benefits to my meals during pregnancy. Incorporating these natural seasonings not only enhanced the taste of my dishes but also provided various nutrients and medicinal properties.

Ginger, for example, was a lifesaver for nausea and morning sickness. A cup of ginger tea in the morning helped soothe my stomach and start the day on a positive note. Fresh ginger added to stir-fries and soups provided a warm, spicy kick and supported digestion.

Turmeric, with its anti-inflammatory properties, became a regular addition to my cooking. I enjoyed making turmeric lattes, blending warm milk with turmeric, honey, and a pinch of black pepper. This golden drink was not only comforting but also provided numerous health benefits. Adding turmeric to rice dishes, soups, and roasted vegetables also boosted their flavor and nutritional value.

Garlic and onions, staples in my kitchen, offered antibacterial and immune-boosting properties. I used them generously in my cooking, from sautéing them as a base for soups and stews to adding raw garlic to salad dressings and dips. These ingredients not only enhanced the taste of my meals but also supported my overall health.

Herbs like parsley, cilantro, and basil added fresh flavors and essential nutrients to my dishes. A handful of chopped parsley sprinkled over roasted vegetables or mixed into quinoa salads brightened up the flavors and added a dose of vitamins A, C, and K. Cilantro was perfect for adding a fresh, zesty note to salsas, tacos, and rice dishes. Fresh basil leaves in salads, pasta dishes, and homemade pesto provided a burst of flavor and beneficial nutrients.

Cinnamon was another spice I frequently used, especially in sweet dishes. Sprinkling cinnamon on my oatmeal, yogurt, or baked apples not only added warmth and sweetness but also helped regulate blood sugar levels. A touch of cinnamon in smoothies or homemade granola bars made them even more delicious and nutritious.

Incorporating herbs and spices into my diet was an enjoyable way to enhance the flavor of my meals while also reaping their health benefits. These natural seasonings made my dishes more exciting and supported my health and well-being during pregnancy.

Superfood Snacks and Recipes

Finding healthy and satisfying snacks was important to me during pregnancy. Incorporating superfoods into my snacks ensured that I was getting the nutrients I needed to support both my health and my baby's development.

One of my favorite snacks was a simple trail mix made with nuts, seeds, and dried fruits. Almonds, walnuts, pumpkin seeds, and dried cranberries mixed together created a delicious and nutrient-dense snack that was easy to take on the go. This mix provided protein, healthy fats, fiber, and a range of vitamins and minerals.

Smoothies were another go-to snack. Blending spinach, berries, Greek yogurt, and a splash of almond milk created a refreshing and nutrient-packed drink. Adding a spoonful of chia seeds or a handful of nuts to the smoothie provided extra protein and healthy fats.

Energy balls made with oats, nut butter, honey, and a variety of add-ins like chia seeds, flaxseeds, and dried fruits were a convenient and tasty snack. These no-bake treats could be made in batches and stored in the fridge, making them perfect for a quick bite when I needed a boost of energy.

Hummus with fresh vegetables became a regular snack in my routine. Carrot sticks, cucumber slices, and bell pepper strips dipped in creamy hummus made for a satisfying and nutritious snack. Hummus, made from chickpeas, tahini, lemon juice, and garlic, provided protein, fiber, and healthy fats.

Greek yogurt parfaits with layers of yogurt, fresh berries, and a sprinkle of granola were another favorite. This snack was not only delicious but also provided a good balance of protein, fiber, and antioxidants.

Homemade kale chips were a fun and crunchy snack. Tossing kale leaves with a bit of olive oil and seasoning, then baking them until crispy, created a nutrient-dense alternative to regular chips. These chips were high in vitamins A, C, and K and made for a guilt-free snack.

Incorporating superfoods into my snacks ensured that I was getting the nutrients I needed to support my health and my baby's development. These snacks were easy to prepare, delicious, and provided a range of health benefits, making them an essential part of my pregnancy diet.

Avocado Toast with Hemp Seeds

Avocado toast became a frequent choice for breakfast or a quick snack. Mashing ripe avocado onto whole grain toast and sprinkling it with hemp seeds added healthy fats, fiber, and protein to my diet. Avocados are rich in folate, potassium, and vitamin C, which are crucial for fetal development and maternal health. Hemp seeds are a great source of plant-based protein and omega-3 fatty acids, supporting brain development in the baby.

Quinoa Salad with Roasted Vegetables

Quinoa became a versatile ingredient in my pregnancy meals, including salads. I often prepared a quinoa salad with roasted vegetables such as bell peppers, zucchini, and cherry tomatoes. Roasting the vegetables enhanced their flavor while adding vitamins A, C, and antioxidants. Quinoa provided protein, fiber, and essential minerals like iron and magnesium, which are vital during pregnancy for energy and muscle function.

Chia Seed Pudding

Chia seed pudding was a delightful and nutritious dessert or snack option. Mixing chia seeds with almond milk and a touch of honey or maple syrup, then letting it sit overnight in the fridge, created a pudding-like texture packed with omega-3 fatty acids, fiber, and protein. Chia seeds are also rich in calcium, magnesium, and antioxidants, supporting bone health and reducing inflammation.

Salmon and Quinoa Patties

Salmon, rich in omega-3 fatty acids, was a cornerstone of my pregnancy diet. I often made salmon and quinoa patties by combining canned salmon, cooked quinoa, diced vegetables, and herbs. These patties were baked until golden brown, providing a delicious source of protein, omega-3s, and essential nutrients like vitamin D and B vitamins. They were easy to prepare in advance and enjoyed warm or cold as a snack or meal.

Yogurt Parfait with Granola and Berries

Yogurt parfaits were a refreshing and nutrient-dense snack that satisfied my sweet cravings. Layering Greek yogurt with fresh berries and a sprinkle of homemade granola provided probiotics, calcium, protein, and antioxidants. Greek yogurt is also high in B vitamins and helps maintain gut health, which is essential during pregnancy for nutrient absorption and immune support.

Edamame Hummus with Whole Grain Crackers
Edamame hummus became a favorite dip for whole grain crackers or vegetable sticks. Edamame, or young soybeans, are packed with protein, fiber, and folate, supporting fetal growth and development. Hummus made from edamame, tahini, lemon juice, and garlic provided a creamy texture and savory flavor, making it a nutritious snack rich in essential nutrients.

Spinach and Feta Stuffed Sweet Potatoes
Sweet potatoes, high in beta-carotene and fiber, were a regular feature in my pregnancy meals. Baking sweet potatoes until tender and stuffing them with sautéed spinach, feta cheese, and a sprinkle of herbs created a satisfying and nutrient-dense dish. Spinach added folate, iron, and vitamins A, C, and K, while feta cheese provide calcium and protein, making this meal beneficial for both me and my baby.

Berry Smoothie with Spinach
Smoothies were a convenient way to incorporate superfoods like berries and spinach into my diet. Mixing fresh or frozen berries with spinach, Greek yogurt, and a splash of almond milk created a delicious and nutrient-packed drink. Berries provided antioxidants,

vitamins, and fiber, while spinach added folate, iron, and other essential nutrients crucial for fetal development and maternal health.

Pumpkin Seed Energy Balls

Energy balls made from pumpkin seeds, oats, nut butter, and honey were a nutritious and energizing snack. Pumpkin seeds are rich in protein, healthy fats, magnesium, and zinc, supporting immune function and fetal development. These no-bake treats were easy to prepare in batches, providing a convenient snack packed with essential nutrients for pregnancy.

Green Smoothie Bowl with Toppings

Green smoothie bowls were a refreshing and nourishing breakfast or snack option. Blending spinach, kale, banana, and avocado with almond milk created a creamy green base. Toppings like chia seeds, sliced fruits, and granola added texture, flavor, and additional nutrients. This bowl was rich in vitamins, minerals, fiber, and healthy fats, supporting overall health during pregnancy.

Incorporating these superfood snacks and recipes into my pregnancy diet ensured that I received a variety of nutrients essential for my health and the development of my baby. These options were not only delicious but also convenient, making it easier to maintain a balanced and nutritious diet throughout pregnancy.

One thing stands out—the profound impact of nutrition on both my well-being and the development of my baby. Eating a diet rich in superfoods has not only nourished me but has also supported the growth and health of my little one. From leafy greens bursting with vitamins to omega-3 packed fatty fish, each superfood has played a vital role in ensuring a healthy pregnancy.

Remember, the choices we make about what we eat during pregnancy can have lasting effects. Incorporating these nutrient-dense superfoods into your diet isn't just about meeting nutritional needs; it's about nurturing yourself and your baby. Whether you enjoy a colorful berry smoothie, indulge in a nutritious yogurt parfait, or savor a hearty quinoa salad, each meal contributes to your journey toward motherhood.

As you go through the joys and challenges of pregnancy, I encourage you to explore these superfoods and discover what works best for you. Experiment with new recipes, embrace wholesome ingredients, and savor the flavors that support your well-being. Your body is doing something incredible—nurturing new life—and by choosing nutrient-rich foods, you're providing the best possible start for your baby.

Chapter 9:

Quick and Nutritious Recipes for Expecting Mothers

Welcome to Chapter 8, a sanctuary of wholesome, nutritious, and straightforward recipes designed with the expecting mother in mind. As the old saying goes, "You are what you eat," so let's nourish your body and growing baby with an array of flavorsome and health-packed meals. Throughout this chapter, we will journey together through various meal types and dietary preferences. From the morning energy boosters to midday satiety promoters, from delightful snack breaks to fulfilling dinners, there is something here for everyone. Each recipe has been carefully curated considering the essential nutrients you and your little one need.

During pregnancy, maintaining a balanced diet is paramount. Not only does it support your health, but it also ensures your baby receives the necessary nutrients for optimal development. This chapter is your guide to quick, nutritious, and delicious meals that cater to different dietary preferences and restrictions. Whether you're a seasoned cook or a kitchen novice, these recipes are designed to be easy to prepare, packed with essential nutrients, and, most importantly, delicious.

We'll cover a variety of meal options, starting with breakfast recipes that promise to kickstart your day with energy and vitality. You'll find lunch and dinner ideas that are both nourishing and satisfying, along with snack options to keep your cravings in check. For those following vegetarian or vegan diets, we've included plant-based recipes rich in essential nutrients. Quick and easy meals will save you time without compromising nutrition, and our healthy desserts will satisfy your sweet tooth in the healthiest way possible.

So, let's go on this culinary journey together, discovering the joy of nourishing your body and baby with each bite.

Breakfast Recipes

Starting your day right is crucial in pregnancy. Our breakfast recipes are beautifully balanced to ensure a steady release of energy throughout the morning while satisfying your taste buds.

One of my favorite go-to breakfast options is overnight oats. They are incredibly versatile and can be prepared the night before, saving you time in the morning. To make a basic version, mix rolled oats with your choice of milk (dairy or plant-based), a dollop of yogurt, and a sprinkle of chia seeds. Let it sit in the fridge overnight. In the morning, top it with fresh fruits like berries or bananas, a handful of nuts for added protein, and a drizzle of honey or maple syrup for sweetness.

Another great option is a veggie-packed egg scramble. Eggs are an excellent source of protein and choline, which is essential for fetal brain development. Start by whisking a couple of eggs in a bowl. In a non-stick pan, sauté some chopped spinach, bell peppers, and tomatoes in a bit of olive oil. Pour in the eggs and scramble until cooked through. Serve with a slice of whole-grain toast for a complete meal.

Smoothies are also a fantastic breakfast choice, especially when you're short on time. Blend together a banana, a handful of spinach, a scoop of Greek yogurt, a tablespoon of almond butter, and some almond milk. This smoothie is not only delicious but also packed with nutrients like calcium, protein, and healthy fats.

For those who prefer a warm breakfast, oatmeal is a classic. Cook rolled oats in milk and top with sliced apples, cinnamon, and a sprinkle of walnuts. This comforting bowl of oatmeal is rich in fiber and keeps you full for longer.

1. Overnight Oats:

Ingredients:
- 1/2 cup rolled oats
- 1/2 cup milk (or plant-based milk)
- 1/2 cup Greek yogurt
- 1 tablespoon chia seeds
- 1 tablespoon honey or maple syrup
- Fresh fruits (berries, bananas, or apples)

Instructions:
- In a jar or bowl, combine oats, milk, Greek yogurt, chia seeds, and honey.
- Mix well and cover.
- Refrigerate overnight.
- In the morning, top with fresh fruits and enjoy.

Nutritional Benefits:

Overnight oats are rich in fiber, which helps prevent constipation, a common pregnancy issue. The addition of Greek yogurt provides protein and probiotics, supporting gut health.

2. Veggie Omelette:

Ingredients:

- 2 eggs
- 1/4 cup chopped bell peppers
- 1/4 cup chopped spinach
- 1/4 cup diced tomatoes
- Salt and pepper to taste
- 1 tablespoon olive oil

Instructions:

- Whisk the eggs in a bowl and season with salt and pepper.
- Heat olive oil in a pan over medium heat.
- Add bell peppers, spinach, and tomatoes. Sauté until soft.
- Pour the eggs over the veggies and cook until the eggs are set.
- Fold the omelette in half and serve.

Nutritional Benefits:

Eggs provide high-quality protein and essential nutrients like choline, which is important for brain development. Vegetables add vitamins and minerals, enhancing the overall nutrient profile

3. Smoothie Bowl:

Ingredients:

- 1 banana
- 1/2 cup frozen berries
- 1/2 cup Greek yogurt
- 1/4 cup milk (or plant-based milk)
- Toppings: granola, nuts, seeds, fresh fruits

Instructions:

- Blend banana, frozen berries, Greek yogurt, and milk until smooth.
- Pour into a bowl.
- Top with granola, nuts, seeds, and fresh fruits.

Nutritional Benefits:

Smoothie bowls are packed with vitamins, antioxidants, and fiber. They are a refreshing and nutrient-dense way to start your day.

Lunch and Dinner Recipes

Prenatal nutrition at its finest! These lunch and dinner recipes offer a perfect blend of proteins, carbohydrates, vitamins, and minerals. With easy-to-follow instructions, you'll be whipping up these healthy meals in no time.

Salads are a great lunch option, and one of my favorites is a quinoa and black bean salad. Cook quinoa according to the package instructions and let it cool. In a large bowl, combine the quinoa with black beans, chopped cherry tomatoes, diced avocado, and corn kernels.

Toss with a lime-cilantro dressing made from lime juice, olive oil, chopped cilantro, and a pinch of salt. This salad is not only refreshing but also rich in protein, fiber, and healthy fats.

For dinner, a hearty vegetable soup can be both comforting and nutritious. Start by sautéing onions, garlic, and celery in a large pot. Add chopped carrots, zucchini, and sweet potatoes, and cook for a few minutes. Pour in vegetable broth and a can of diced tomatoes. Let it simmer until the vegetables are tender. Season with herbs like thyme and rosemary, and add a handful of kale towards the end of cooking. This soup is packed with vitamins and minerals, making it a perfect dinner choice.

Another delicious dinner option is a baked salmon with roasted vegetables. Salmon is a great source of omega-3 fatty acids, which are crucial for fetal brain development. Season a salmon filet with salt, pepper, and a squeeze of lemon juice. Bake in the oven at 375°F for about 20 minutes. Serve with a side of roasted vegetables like Brussels sprouts, carrots, and bell peppers, drizzled with olive oil and sprinkled with herbs.

For a vegetarian option, try a lentil and vegetable stir-fry. Cook lentils according to the package instructions. In a large pan, sauté chopped onions, garlic, and bell peppers in olive oil. Add cooked lentils, a handful of spinach, and a splash of soy sauce. Stir-fry for a few minutes until everything is heated through. Serve over brown rice or quinoa for a complete meal.

1. Quinoa Salad:

Ingredients:

- 1 cup cooked quinoa
- 1/2 cup cherry tomatoes, halved
- 1/2 cucumber, diced
- 1/4 cup red onion, diced
- 1/4 cup feta cheese, crumbled
- 2 tablespoons olive oil
- 1 tablespoon lemon juice
- Salt and pepper to taste

Instructions:

- In a large bowl, combine cooked quinoa, cherry tomatoes, cucumber, red onion, and feta cheese.
- Drizzle with olive oil and lemon juice.
- Season with salt and pepper.
- Toss to combine and serve.

Nutritional Benefits:

Quinoa is a complete protein, providing all nine essential amino acids. It's also rich in fiber, iron, and magnesium, supporting overall health during pregnancy.

2. Chicken and Vegetable Stir-Fry:

Ingredients:

- 2 chicken breasts, sliced
- 1 cup broccoli florets
- 1 red bell pepper, sliced
- 1 carrot, julienned
- 2 tablespoons soy sauce
- 1 tablespoon olive oil
- 1 teaspoon ginger, minced
- 2 cloves garlic, minced

Instructions:

- Heat olive oil in a large pan over medium heat.
- Add chicken and cook until browned.
- Add ginger and garlic, sauté for 1 minute.
- Add broccoli, bell pepper, and carrot. Cook until vegetables are tender.
- Stir in soy sauce and cook for another 2 minutes.
- Serve with brown rice or quinoa.

Nutritional Benefits: This stir-fry is packed with protein from the chicken and a variety of vitamins and minerals from the vegetables. It's a balanced meal that supports both maternal health and fetal development.

3. Lentil Soup:

Ingredients:

- 1 cup lentils, rinsed
- 1 onion, diced
- 2 carrots, diced
- 2 celery stalks, diced
- 4 cups vegetable broth
- 1 can diced tomatoes
- 1 teaspoon cumin
- 1 teaspoon turmeric
- Salt and pepper to taste

Instructions:

- In a large pot, sauté onion, carrots, and celery until softened.
- Add lentils, vegetable broth, diced tomatoes, cumin, and turmeric.
- Bring to a boil, then reduce heat and simmer for 30 minutes or until lentils are tender.
- Season with salt and pepper before serving.

Nutritional Benefits:

Lentils are a great source of plant-based protein, fiber, and iron, making this soup a hearty and nutritious option for expecting mothers.

<u>Snack Recipes</u>

Snacking is essential during pregnancy to keep energy levels up and manage hunger between meals. Here are some quick and nutritious snack ideas.

1. Energy Balls:

Ingredients:

- 1 cup rolled oats
- 1/2 cup peanut butter
- 1/4 cup honey
- 1/4 cup dark chocolate chips
- 1/4 cup flaxseeds

Instructions:

- In a bowl, mix all ingredients until well combined.
- Roll the mixture into small balls.
- Refrigerate for 30 minutes before serving.

Nutritional Benefits:

Energy balls are rich in healthy fats, fiber, and protein, providing a quick energy boost and satisfying hunger.

2. Hummus and Veggies:

Ingredients:

- 1 can chickpeas, drained and rinsed
- 1/4 cup tahini
- 1/4 cup olive oil
- 1 lemon, juiced
- 2 cloves garlic, minced
- Salt to taste
- Fresh vegetables (carrots, celery, bell peppers) for dipping

Instructions:

- In a food processor, blend chickpeas, tahini, olive oil, lemon juice, garlic, and salt until smooth.
- Serve with fresh vegetables for dipping.

Nutritional Benefits:

Hummus is high in protein and healthy fats, while fresh vegetables provide vitamins, minerals, and fiber, making this a nutritious and satisfying snack.

3. Greek Yogurt with Honey and Nuts:

Ingredients:

1 cup Greek yogurt

1 tablespoon honey

1/4 cup mixed nuts (almonds, walnuts, pistachios)

Instructions:

- In a bowl, combine Greek yogurt, honey, and mixed nuts.
- Mix well and serve.

Nutritional Benefits:

Greek yogurt is a great source of protein and probiotics, supporting gut health. Nuts add healthy fats, protein, and essential nutrients like magnesium and vitamin E.

Vegetarian and Vegan Options

For those following a vegetarian or vegan diet, it's important to ensure adequate intake of essential nutrients. Here are some delicious plant-based recipes.

1. Lentil and Vegetable Stew:

Ingredients:

- 1 cup lentils, rinsed
- 1 zucchini, diced
- 1 bell pepper, diced
- 1 sweet potato, diced
- 1 onion, diced
- 4 cups vegetable broth
- 1 can diced tomatoes
- 1 teaspoon thyme
- 1 teaspoon rosemary
- Salt and pepper to taste

Instructions:

In a large pot, sauté onion until softened.

- Add zucchini, bell pepper, sweet potato, lentils, vegetable broth, diced tomatoes, thyme, and rosemary.
- Bring to a boil, then reduce heat and simmer for 30 minutes or until lentils and vegetables are tender.
- Season with salt and pepper before serving.

Nutritional Benefits:

This stew is rich in plant-based protein, fiber, vitamins, and minerals, making it a hearty and nutritious option for pregnant women.

2. Quinoa and Black Bean Salad:

Ingredients:

- 1 cup cooked quinoa
- 1 can black beans, drained and rinsed
- 1 cup corn kernels
- 1 red bell pepper, diced
- 1/4 cup chopped cilantro
- 2 tablespoons olive oil
- 1 tablespoon lime juice
- Salt and pepper to taste

Instructions:

- In a large bowl, combine cooked quinoa, black beans, corn, bell pepper, and cilantro.

- Drizzle with olive oil and lime juice.
- Season with salt and pepper.
- Toss to combine and serve.

Nutritional Benefits:

Quinoa and black beans provide a complete protein source, along with fiber, iron, and folate. This salad is a nutritious and satisfying meal option.

Quick and Easy Meals

Sometimes, you need meals that are quick to prepare but still nutritious. Here are some easy recipes that can be made in no time.

1. One-Pot Pasta:

Ingredients:

- 8 oz whole wheat pasta
- 1 can diced tomatoes
- 2 cups vegetable broth
- 1 zucchini, sliced
- 1 bell pepper, sliced
- 1 onion, diced
- 2 cloves garlic, minced
- 1 tablespoon olive oil
- 1 teaspoon oregano
- Salt and pepper to taste

Instructions:

- In a large pot, heat olive oil over medium heat.
- Add onion and garlic, sauté until softened.
- Add zucchini and bell pepper, cook for 3 minutes.
- Add pasta, diced tomatoes, vegetable broth, oregano, salt, and pepper.
- Bring to a boil, then reduce heat and simmer until pasta is cooked and liquid is absorbed, about 15 minutes.
- Serve immediately.

Nutritional Benefits:

This one-pot pasta is a balanced meal with whole grains, vegetables, and healthy fats, providing essential nutrients in a quick and convenient dish.

2. 30-Minute Chicken Stir-Fry:

Ingredients:

- 2 chicken breasts, sliced
- 1 cup broccoli florets
- 1 red bell pepper, sliced
- 1 carrot, julienned
- 2 tablespoons soy sauce
- 1 tablespoon olive oil
- 1 teaspoon ginger, minced
- 2 cloves garlic, minced

Instructions:

- Heat olive oil in a large pan over medium heat.
- Add chicken and cook until browned.
- Add ginger and garlic, sauté for 1 minute.

- Add broccoli, bell pepper, and carrot. Cook until vegetables are tender.
- Stir in soy sauce and cook for another 2 minutes.
- Serve with brown rice or quinoa.

Nutritional Benefits:

This stir-fry is packed with protein from the chicken and a variety of vitamins and minerals from the vegetables. It's a balanced meal that supports both maternal health and fetal development.

Healthy Desserts

Satisfy your sweet tooth with these healthy dessert options that are both delicious and nutritious.

1. Fruit Salad with Honey-Lime Dressing:

Ingredients:
- 1 cup strawberries, sliced
- 1 cup blueberries
- 1 cup pineapple, diced
- 1 cup mango, diced
- 1 tablespoon honey
- 1 tablespoon lime juice

Instructions:
- In a large bowl, combine strawberries, blueberries, pineapple, and mango.
- Drizzle with honey and lime juice.
- Toss to combine and serve.

Nutritional Benefits:

Fruit salad is rich in vitamins, antioxidants, and fiber, making it a refreshing and nutritious dessert option.

2. Greek Yogurt Parfait:

Ingredients:

- 1 cup Greek yogurt
- 1 tablespoon honey
- 1/4 cup granola
- Fresh berries (strawberries, blueberries, raspberries)

Instructions:

- In a glass or bowl, layer Greek yogurt, honey, granola, and fresh berries.
- Repeat layers until all ingredients are used.
- Serve immediately.

Nutritional Benefits:

Greek yogurt parfaits are rich in protein, probiotics, and antioxidants, making them a healthy and satisfying dessert choice.

Well done on nourishing yourself and your baby with these quick and nutritious recipes! Remember, a varied diet combining the recipes from this chapter is key to meeting all your prenatal nutritional needs. These meals are designed to support your health and your baby's development, providing you with the energy and nutrients necessary for this special time in your life.

From breakfast to dessert, each recipe offers a balanced mix of essential nutrients tailored to the needs of expecting mothers. By incorporating these delicious and healthy options into your daily routine, you're taking an important step towards ensuring a healthy pregnancy and a strong foundation for your baby's growth.

Happy cooking, and enjoy every bite of this beautiful journey!

Chapter 9:

Postpartum Nutrition: Rebuilding and Replenishing After Birth

When I started this incredible journey of motherhood, I quickly realized that the postpartum period brought its own unique set of challenges and needs. After months of nurturing and nourishing my body to support my growing baby, the time had come to focus on my own recovery and well-being. The transition from pregnancy to motherhood was both joyful and overwhelming, and it became clear that my body required special attention to heal and thrive.

In this chapter, I will share the wisdom and insights I gained about postpartum nutrition—knowledge that became a cornerstone of my recovery. The days and weeks following childbirth are a crucial time for rebuilding and replenishing our bodies. We need to restore depleted nutrient and energy stores, support lactation, and promote overall healing. This period isn't just about bouncing back; it's about nurturing ourselves as we nurture our newborns.

We will explore the specific nutritional needs that arise after giving birth and discover the foods and practices that can best support our bodies during this time. From rebuilding muscle and strength to aiding in uterine shrinkage and managing postpartum bleeding, proper nutrition plays a pivotal role. Additionally, we'll delve into the relationship between breastfeeding and nutrition, understanding how what we eat can enhance milk production and quality.

To make this journey easier, I'll share practical meal ideas, snacks, and smoothie recipes that are both nutritious and easy to prepare. We'll also look at how meal delivery services can be a lifesaver for busy new moms. Moreover, we'll emphasize the importance of self-care and the profound connection between nutrition and mental health, providing strategies to build a supportive network around us.

Finally, I'll present a comprehensive 30-day meal plan designed to meet the unique nutritional demands of the postpartum period. This chapter is intended to be a guide, offering support and encouragement as we navigate this new and beautiful phase of life, ensuring that we care for ourselves as diligently as we care for our little ones.

Postpartum Nutritional Needs

After childbirth, your body undergoes significant changes and requires ample nutrition to recover and thrive. The immediate postpartum period is marked by the need to replenish depleted nutrients, support lactation, and promote healing and recovery. Let's delve into the specific nutritional requirements during this critical phase.

Replenishing Depleted Nutrients:

Iron: During childbirth, many women experience blood loss, which can lead to a reduction in iron levels. Iron is crucial for producing hemoglobin, which carries oxygen in the blood. Low iron levels can result in postpartum anemia, characterized by fatigue, weakness, and dizziness. To replenish iron, include foods such as lean meats, fish, beans, spinach, and fortified cereals in your diet. Pairing iron-rich foods with vitamin C sources, like citrus fruits or bell peppers, can enhance iron absorption.

Calcium: Pregnancy and breastfeeding can deplete your calcium stores. Calcium is vital for bone health and muscle function. To maintain strong bones and teeth, consume calcium-rich foods such as dairy products (milk, cheese, and yogurt), fortified plant-based milk (almond, soy), leafy green vegetables, and nuts. If you have difficulty meeting your calcium needs through diet alone, consider a calcium supplement after consulting with your healthcare provider.

Vitamin D: This nutrient aids in calcium absorption and supports immune function. Vitamin D deficiency is common, especially in regions with limited sunlight. Sun exposure can help your body produce vitamin D, but it's also important to include dietary sources like fatty fish (salmon, mackerel), fortified milk, and egg yolks. If needed, a vitamin D supplement can ensure adequate levels.

Omega-3 Fatty Acids: These essential fats, particularly DHA, are important for brain health and reducing inflammation. Omega-3s can be found in fatty fish (like salmon and sardines), flaxseeds, chia seeds, and walnuts. If you don't consume fish regularly, consider taking a fish oil supplement or an algae-based omega-3 supplement if you're vegetarian or vegan.

Protein: Protein is necessary for tissue repair and muscle recovery. Include a variety of protein sources such as lean meats, poultry, fish, eggs, dairy, beans, lentils, and nuts. Adequate protein intake can help rebuild muscle strength and support overall recovery.

Supporting Lactation and Breastfeeding:

Breastfeeding increases your nutritional needs significantly. Producing breast milk requires an additional 500 calories per day on average. These extra calories should come from nutrient-dense foods that provide the vitamins and minerals necessary for both you and your baby. A balanced diet rich in fruits, vegetables, whole grains, lean proteins, and healthy fats supports milk production and ensures your breast milk is rich in essential nutrients.

Promoting Healing and Recovery:

Postpartum recovery involves healing from childbirth, which can be aided by certain foods and nutrients.

Antioxidant-rich foods: Fruits and vegetables high in antioxidants, such as berries, spinach, and sweet potatoes, help reduce inflammation and promote healing.

Collagen: Foods high in collagen, like bone broth and chicken, can support tissue repair and improve skin elasticity, aiding in the healing of perineal tears or cesarean sections.

Zinc: This mineral plays a role in immune function and wound healing. Foods like meat, shellfish, legumes, and seeds are good sources of zinc.

Focusing on nutrient-dense foods that replenish iron, calcium, vitamin D, omega-3 fatty acids, and protein can significantly aid postpartum recovery. Additionally, supporting lactation through a balanced diet ensures both you and your baby receive the necessary nutrients. Prioritizing these nutritional needs will help you recover more quickly and feel more energized as you embark on your journey into motherhood.

Nourishing Your Body

The postpartum period is a time for your body to heal and regain strength after the physical demands of pregnancy and childbirth. Proper nourishment is essential to support this recovery process, including rebuilding muscle, supporting uterine shrinkage, and managing postpartum bleeding. Here's how to focus on these key areas effectively.

Rebuilding Muscle and Strength:

Protein: Protein is fundamental for muscle repair and recovery. Aim to include a variety of protein sources in your daily diet, such as lean meats, poultry, fish, eggs, dairy products, beans, lentils, and nuts. For instance, starting your day with a breakfast that includes eggs or Greek yogurt can provide a good protein boost.

Complex Carbohydrates: These provide sustained energy, which is crucial for new mothers who are often sleep-deprived and fatigued. Whole grains like oats, quinoa, brown rice, and whole wheat bread are excellent options. Including complex carbohydrates in your meals helps maintain energy levels throughout the day.

Healthy Fats: Fats are not only a source of energy but also important for absorbing fat-soluble vitamins (A, D, E, K) and supporting overall health. Incorporate healthy fats from sources like avocados, nuts, seeds, olive oil, and fatty fish into your diet. A salad with avocado and a drizzle of olive oil, or a handful of almonds as a snack, can boost your healthy fat intake.

Supporting Uterine Shrinkage and Vaginal Healing:

Hydration: Staying well-hydrated is crucial for many bodily functions, including supporting uterine contractions that help shrink the uterus back to its pre-pregnancy size. Aim to drink at least 8-10 glasses of water daily. Herbal teas and broths can also contribute to your hydration needs.

Anti-Inflammatory Foods:

 Inflammation can slow down the healing process, so including anti-inflammatory foods in your diet can be beneficial. Turmeric, ginger, garlic, and berries are known for their anti-inflammatory properties. Adding a bit of fresh ginger to your smoothies or sipping on turmeric tea can help reduce inflammation.

Collagen-Rich Foods

 Collagen is a protein that supports skin elasticity and tissue repair. Bone broth, which is rich in collagen, can be easily incorporated into soups or stews. Chicken, particularly with the skin, also provides collagen, which can aid in the healing of tissues after childbirth.

Iron-Rich Foods: Postpartum bleeding, or lochia, can last for several weeks, leading to iron loss. To prevent iron deficiency, include iron-rich foods in your diet. Red meat, poultry, fish, beans, lentils, spinach, and fortified cereals are excellent sources. Combining these with vitamin C-rich foods can enhance iron absorption. For example, a spinach salad with strawberries or bell peppers can be both nutritious and beneficial for iron levels.

Vitamin C: This vitamin not only boosts your immune system but also improves iron absorption, which is essential during the postpartum period. Citrus fruits, strawberries, bell peppers, and broccoli are all high in vitamin C. Starting your day with a glass of orange juice or adding bell peppers to your meals can help meet your vitamin C needs.

Fiber: Constipation is a common issue postpartum, especially if you've had a cesarean section or are taking iron supplements. High-fiber foods like fruits, vegetables, whole grains, and legumes can help prevent constipation and promote regular bowel movements. A breakfast of oatmeal topped with berries and a sprinkle of flaxseeds can provide a good fiber boost.

Nourishing your body after childbirth involves a balanced intake of proteins, complex carbohydrates, healthy fats, and essential vitamins and minerals. These nutrients support muscle rebuilding, uterine shrinkage, vaginal healing, and the management of postpartum bleeding. By focusing on these dietary elements, you can enhance your recovery, regain strength, and better manage the physical demands of motherhood. Remember, every meal and snack is an opportunity to nourish your body and support your postpartum journey.

Breastfeeding and Nutrition

Breastfeeding is a beautiful and natural way to nourish your baby, but it also places significant nutritional demands on your body. Understanding these demands and meeting them through a balanced diet is crucial for both your health and your baby's development. This section will cover the nutritional requirements for lactation, foods that support milk production, and common breastfeeding challenges with their solutions.

Nutritional Requirements for Lactation:

Calories: Breastfeeding mothers need an additional 500 calories per day to support milk production. These extra calories should come from nutrient-dense foods rather than empty calories. Focus on whole grains, lean proteins, healthy fats, and plenty of fruits and vegetables.

Hydration: Adequate hydration is essential for maintaining a healthy milk supply. Aim to drink at least 8-10 glasses of water per day. Herbal teas and broths can also help keep you hydrated. Remember to drink a glass of water each time you nurse to stay properly hydrated.

Vitamins and Minerals: Key nutrients for lactation include calcium, iron, vitamin D, and B vitamins. A varied diet rich in these nutrients will support both you and your baby's health. For example, include dairy products or fortified plant-based milk for calcium, lean meats and leafy greens for iron, fatty fish for vitamin D, and whole grains for B vitamins.

Foods That Support Milk Production:

Oats: Oats are a well-known galactagogue, meaning they can help increase milk production. Start your day with a bowl of oatmeal or add oats to smoothies and baked goods.

Fenugreek: This herb is commonly used to boost milk supply. It can be taken as a supplement or brewed into tea. However, consult with your healthcare provider before starting any new supplements.

Garlic: Garlic is believed to enhance the flavor of breast milk and may encourage your baby to nurse more, thereby increasing milk supply. Incorporate garlic into your cooking, such as in soups, stews, and stir-fries.

Leafy Greens: Spinach, kale, and other leafy greens are rich in phytoestrogens, which may support milk production. Include a variety of leafy greens in your diet through salads, smoothies, and side dishes.

Nuts and Seeds: Almonds, flaxseeds, and chia seeds provide healthy fats and proteins that support lactation. Snack on a handful of nuts or add seeds to your yogurt and smoothies for an extra boost.

Common Breastfeeding Challenges and Solutions:

Low Milk Supply: If you're concerned about low milk supply, ensure you're nursing or pumping frequently, as milk production works on a supply-and-demand basis. Additionally, staying hydrated and consuming galactagogues like oats and fenugreek can help. Consult a lactation consultant for personalized advice.

Sore Nipples: Sore nipples are a common issue, especially in the early days of breastfeeding. Ensure your baby is latching correctly, as an improper latch can cause pain and damage to the nipples. Use nipple creams or ointments, and allow your nipples to air dry after nursing.

Breast Engorgement: Engorgement can be painful and make it difficult for your baby to latch. To relieve engorgement, try expressing some milk before nursing to soften the breast. Applying warm compresses before feeding and cold compresses afterward can also help reduce swelling and discomfort.

Mastitis: This breast infection can cause fever, pain, and redness. If you suspect mastitis, continue breastfeeding or pumping to keep the milk flowing, as this can help clear the infection. Apply warm compresses and ensure proper rest. If symptoms persist, seek medical treatment as antibiotics may be necessary.

Breastfeeding requires a well-balanced diet rich in essential nutrients and adequate hydration to support both you and your baby. Incorporating foods that boost milk production and addressing common breastfeeding challenges can make the experience more enjoyable and less stressful. Remember, each mother's breastfeeding journey is unique, and seeking support from healthcare providers and lactation consultants can be incredibly beneficial.

Postpartum Meal Ideas and Planning

Eating well after childbirth is crucial for your recovery and for providing the necessary nutrients for breastfeeding. However, the demands of caring for a newborn can make meal preparation challenging. This section offers easy and nutritious meal prep ideas, snack options, and smoothie recipes, along with information on meal delivery and preparation services.

Easy and Nutritious Meal Prep Ideas:

Batch Cooking: Prepare large batches of meals that can be frozen in individual portions. This way, you have healthy, ready-to-eat meals on hand. Examples include soups, stews, casseroles, and chili. For instance, a big pot of vegetable and lentil soup can provide several servings that are easy to reheat.

Sheet Pan Meals: These are convenient and require minimal cleanup. Simply arrange your protein (like chicken or fish) and vegetables (such as bell peppers, broccoli, and sweet potatoes) on a baking sheet, drizzle with olive oil, season, and bake. You can make a variety of combinations to keep meals interesting.

Slow Cooker Recipes: Slow cookers can be a lifesaver for busy new moms. Ingredients can be prepped in the morning and cooked throughout the day. Dishes like pulled chicken, beef stew, and vegetable curry are nutritious and effortless.

Nutritious Snack Options:

Greek Yogurt with Honey and Nuts: This snack is rich in protein, healthy fats, and probiotics. The nuts add a satisfying crunch and additional nutrients.

Carrot Sticks with Hummus: Carrots are packed with vitamins, and hummus provides protein and fiber. This combination is both refreshing and filling.

Fruit and Nut Butter: Apples or bananas paired with almond or peanut butter make a quick and nutritious snack. The combination of carbohydrates, protein, and healthy fats provides sustained energy.

Trail Mix: Create your own trail mix with a mix of nuts, seeds, dried fruits, and a bit of dark chocolate. This is an excellent on-the-go snack that's both satisfying and nutritious.

Smoothie Recipes:

Green Smoothie: Blend together spinach, banana, almond milk, chia seeds, and a scoop of protein powder for a nutrient-dense smoothie. This is an excellent way to get your greens without the taste being overwhelming.

Berry Blast: Combine mixed berries (strawberries, blueberries, and raspberries), Greek yogurt, honey, and a splash of orange juice. This smoothie is rich in antioxidants and protein.

Tropical Delight: Blend mango, pineapple, coconut milk, and a handful of spinach for a refreshing, tropical-flavored smoothie. Adding a scoop of collagen powder can provide additional protein and support tissue repair.

Meal Delivery and Preparation Services:

Meal Kits: Services like Blue Apron, HelloFresh, and Sun Basket delivery meal kits with pre-measured ingredients and recipes. This can save time on grocery shopping and meal prep, making it easier to cook nutritious meals at home.

Prepared Meal Delivery: Companies such as Freshly and Daily Harvest offer fully prepared meals that are delivered to your door. These meals just need to be heated, providing a convenient option for those particularly busy days.

Local Services: Many local businesses and personal chefs offer meal prep services tailored to your dietary needs. This personalized service can be particularly helpful in ensuring you're meeting your nutritional goals.

Meal Planning Tips:

Weekly Planning: Set aside time each week to plan your meals. Create a grocery list based on your meal plan to ensure you have all the ingredients you need. This can help reduce last-minute stress and ensure you're eating balanced meals.

Flexible Plans: Be flexible with your meal plans and allow for changes as needed. Sometimes plans don't go as expected, and that's okay. Have a few backup meal options that are easy to prepare, like pasta with marinara sauce or a simple stir-fry.

Involve Your Support System: Don't hesitate to ask for help from family and friends. They can assist with grocery shopping, meal prep, or even bringing over a meal. Having a support system can make a big difference in managing postpartum nutrition.

Planning and preparing nutritious meals after childbirth can be made easier with batch cooking, convenient recipes, and healthy snacks. Utilizing meal delivery services can also provide much-needed support during this busy time. By prioritizing meal planning and involving your support system, you can ensure that you're nourishing your body effectively during the postpartum period.

Self-Care and Nutrition

The postpartum period is not only a time for physical recovery but also a critical phase for mental and emotional well-being. Prioritizing self-care and understanding the link between nutrition and mental health can make a significant difference in how you feel and cope during this time. This section emphasizes the importance of self-care, explores the connection between nutrition and mental health, and suggests ways to build a support network.

Prioritizing Self-Care

Rest and Sleep: One of the most crucial aspects of self-care during the postpartum period is getting enough rest. Sleep deprivation is common for new mothers, but it's essential to rest whenever possible. Nap when the baby naps, and don't hesitate to ask for help with nighttime feedings or household chores.

Hydration: Staying hydrated is vital for both physical and mental health. Dehydration can lead to fatigue, headaches, and difficulty concentrating. Make it a habit to drink water throughout the day. Keep a water bottle within reach, especially while breastfeeding.

Mindfulness and Relaxation: Incorporate relaxation techniques such as deep breathing, meditation, or gentle yoga into your daily routine. These practices can help reduce stress and anxiety, improve mood, and enhance overall well-being. Even a few minutes of mindfulness can make a significant difference.

Pampering Yourself: Take time to pamper yourself, whether it's a warm bath, a massage, or simply reading a book you enjoy. Small acts of self-care can boost your mood and provide a sense of normalcy and comfort during the postpartum period.

Nutrition and Mental Health

Omega-3 Fatty Acids: Omega-3s, particularly DHA, play a crucial role in brain health and mood regulation. Studies have shown that omega-3 supplementation can reduce symptoms of postpartum depression. Include fatty fish like salmon, flaxseeds, and walnuts in your diet to boost your omega-3 intake.

B Vitamins: B vitamins, especially B6, B12, and folate, are essential for brain function and can influence mood and energy levels. Whole grains, leafy greens, beans, and eggs are excellent sources of B vitamins. A balanced diet that includes these foods can help support mental health.

Magnesium: Magnesium is known for its calming effects and ability to reduce anxiety and improve sleep quality. Foods rich in magnesium include dark leafy greens, nuts, seeds, and whole grains. Incorporating these into your meals can help maintain stable mental health.

Probiotics: Gut health is closely linked to mental health, and probiotics can play a role in maintaining a healthy gut microbiome. Yogurt, kefir, sauerkraut, and other fermented foods are good sources of probiotics. A healthy gut can positively impact your mood and overall well-being.

Building a Support Network:

Family and Friends: Don't hesitate to lean on your family and friends for support. They can help with household tasks, provide emotional support, or simply be there to listen. Sharing your feelings and experiences with loved ones can alleviate feelings of isolation and stress.

Support Groups: Joining a postpartum support group can connect you with other new mothers who are experiencing similar challenges. These groups can provide valuable advice, encouragement, and a sense of community. Many hospitals and community centers offer support groups, both in-person and online.

Professional Help: If you're struggling with postpartum depression or anxiety, seeking professional help is crucial. A therapist or counselor specializing in postpartum issues can provide the support and treatment you need. Don't hesitate to reach out to your healthcare provider for recommendations.

Self-Compassion: Be kind to yourself and recognize that adjusting to motherhood takes time. It's normal to feel overwhelmed, and it's important to give yourself grace. Celebrate small victories and be patient with yourself as you navigate this new chapter.

Prioritizing self-care and understanding the impact of nutrition on mental health are essential components of postpartum recovery. By incorporating nutrient-dense foods that support mental well-being, practicing relaxation techniques, and building a strong support network, you can enhance your overall health and resilience during this transformative period. Remember, taking care of yourself is not only beneficial for you but also for your baby, as a healthy and happy mother is better equipped to provide the care and love that your child needs.

Postpartum Nutrition Plan

A comprehensive postpartum nutrition plan can help you stay on track with your dietary goals. Here's a 30-day meal plan designed to meet your postnatal nutritional needs:

Week 1:

- ✓ Breakfast: Overnight oats with chia seeds and fresh berries.
- ✓ Lunch: Quinoa salad with mixed greens and grilled chicken.
- ✓ Dinner: Baked salmon with sweet potato wedges and steamed broccoli.
- ✓ Snacks: Greek yogurt with honey and walnuts; carrot sticks with hummus.

Week 2:

- ✓ Breakfast: Scrambled eggs with spinach and whole-grain toast.
- ✓ Lunch: Whole-grain wrap with hummus, avocado, and turkey slices.
- ✓ Dinner: Stir-fry with tofu, mixed vegetables, and brown rice.
- ✓ Snacks: Fresh fruit with nut butter; trail mix with nuts, seeds, and dried fruit.

Week 3:

- ✓ Breakfast: Greek yogurt parfait with granola and honey.
- ✓ Lunch: Lentil soup with whole-grain bread.
- ✓ Dinner: Spaghetti squash with marinara sauce and turkey meatballs.
- ✓ Snacks: Energy balls made with oats, almond butter, and dark chocolate chips; green smoothie.

Week 4:

- ✓ Breakfast: Smoothie made with spinach, banana, almond milk, chia seeds, and peanut butter.

✓ Lunch: Quinoa salad with mixed greens, cherry tomatoes, cucumbers, and grilled chicken.

✓ Dinner: Baked salmon with sweet potato wedges and steamed broccoli.

✓ Snacks: Greek yogurt with honey and walnuts; carrot sticks with hummus.

Meal Preparation and Planning Tips

- Batch Cooking: Prepare large batches of meals and freeze them in portion sizes for easy reheating.

- Grocery List: Keep a running grocery list of essentials to ensure you always have healthy ingredients on hand.

- Healthy Snacks: Stock up on healthy snacks like nuts, seeds, fresh fruits, and yogurt to curb hunger between meals.

- Flexible Plan: Be flexible with your meal plan and allow for occasional treats. Balance is key.

- Encouragement for a Healthy Postpartum Journey:

- Remember, taking care of yourself is essential for taking care of your baby. Prioritize your nutrition, rest, and mental health, and don't hesitate to seek help when needed. You're doing an incredible job, and with a little planning and support, you can navigate this postpartum period with confidence and grace.

The postpartum period is a time of significant change and adjustment. Proper nutrition can make a substantial difference in your recovery, energy levels, and overall well-being. By understanding your nutritional needs, nourishing your body, supporting breastfeeding, planning meals, and prioritizing self-care, you can set the foundation for a healthy, happy postpartum journey.

Congratulations on this new chapter of motherhood. Embrace it with the knowledge that you're equipped with the tools and resources to thrive. Your dedication to your health and well-being is a gift to both yourself and your baby.

Conclusion

As I reach the end of this journey with you through "Prenatal Nutrition: A Self-Care Approach to Nourishing Your Body and Baby," I am filled with immense gratitude and excitement for the path ahead. Together, we've explored the vital nutrients essential for a healthy pregnancy, discovered the power of superfoods, and learned how to create quick, nutritious meals that cater to our unique needs. This book was written with you in mind, to empower and equip you with the knowledge to make the best choices for you and your precious baby.

Pregnancy is a remarkable and transformative time. It's a journey of growth, not just for your baby, but for you as well. Nourishing your body with the right foods is an act of love, a way to support both your health and the development of your baby. Each chapter in this book has provided a piece of the puzzle, helping you build a foundation of wellness that will benefit you long after your baby is born.

Reflecting on the content we've covered, I hope you feel a sense of empowerment. Whether it was understanding the importance of leafy greens, enjoying the antioxidant boost from berries, or mastering quick and easy meal prep, every step has been a testament to your commitment to health and well-being. You've embraced the journey, celebrated the small victories, and made choices that honor your body and baby.

Pregnancy is a time of incredible change and growth, both physically and emotionally. The nourishment you provide your body not only supports your baby's development but also fortifies your own health and well-being. Each chapter of this book has been designed to equip you with the knowledge and tools to make the best choices for you and your baby.

From leafy greens rich in essential vitamins to the healing power of postpartum nutrition, every bit of information is a step toward a healthier, happier you.

But beyond the science and recipes, this journey is about embracing the joy and wonder of motherhood. It's about celebrating the small victories, like making a delicious, nutrient-packed smoothie or finding the perfect meal that satisfies both cravings and nutritional needs. It's about recognizing the strength within you as you nourish your body and nurture your growing baby

As you move forward, remember that this is just the beginning. Continue to prioritize your health, experiment with new recipes, and listen to your body's needs. Surround yourself with a supportive community, seek advice when needed, and never underestimate the power of self-care. Your well-being is the cornerstone of your baby's health and happiness.

Motherhood is a journey filled with moments of joy, challenge, and profound love. Trust in yourself, celebrate your strength, and know that you are doing an extraordinary job. Embrace this new chapter with confidence and joy, knowing that every step you take towards better nutrition is a step towards a brighter future for you and your baby. Here's to a healthy, happy, and nourishing journey ahead. You've got this!